MENSTRUAL DISORDERS AND MENOPAUSE

MENSTRUAL DISORDERS AND MENOPAUSE

Biological, Psychological, and Cultural Research

Linda R. Gannon

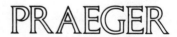

PRAEGER

PRAEGER SPECIAL STUDIES • PRAEGER SCIENTIFIC

New York • Philadelphia • Eastbourne, UK
Toronto • Hong Kong • Tokyo • Sydney

Library of Congress Cataloging in Publication Data

Gannon, Linda.
    Menstrual disorders and menopause.

    Bibliography: p.
    Includes indexes.
    1. Menstruation disorders. 2. Menopause.
I. Title. [DNLM: 1. Menopause. 2. Menstruation
Disorders. WP 550 G198m]
RG161.G35 1985   618.1'72   85-3629
ISBN 0-03-003878-2 (alk. paper)
ISBN 0-03-063243-9 (pbk. : alk. paper)

Published in 1985 by Praeger Publishers
CBS Educational and Professional Publishing, a Division of CBS Inc.
521 Fifth Avenue, New York, NY 10175 USA

© 1985 by Praeger Publishers

56789 052 987654321

Printed in the United States of America on acid-free paper

INTERNATIONAL OFFICES

Orders from outside the United States should be sent to the appropriate address listed below. Orders from areas not listed below should be placed through CBS International Publishing. 383 Madison Ave., New York, NY 10175 USA

Australia, New Zealand
Holt Saunders. Pty. Ltd.. 9 Waltham St.. Artarmon. N.S.W. 2064, Sydney. Australia

Canada
Holt. Rinehart & Winston of Canada. 55 Horner Ave.. Toronto. Ontario, Canada M8Z 4X6

Europe, the Middle East, & Africa
Holt Saunders. Ltd.. 1 St. Anne's Road. Eastbourne. East Sussex, England BN21 3UN

Japan
Holt Saunders. Ltd.. Ichibancho Central Building. 22-1 Ichibancho. 3rd Floor, Chiyodaku, Tokyo, Japan

Hong Kong, Southeast Asia
Holt Saunders Asia. Ltd.. 10 Fl. Intercontinental Plaza. 94 Granville Road, Tsim Sha Tsui East. Kowloon, Hong Kong

Manuscript submissions should be sent to the Editorial Director, Praeger Publishers, 521 Fifth Avenue, New York, NY 10175 USA

Contents

Introduction

> . . . when children cease to be altogether desirable,
> women cease to be altogether necessary.

Virginia Woolf, 1929, p. 116

Ever since Aristotle described woman as a mutilated man, various versions of the "biology as destiny" theme have been applied to woman, rendering her inferior to man who was believed to be guided by his intellect. By the nineteenth century, these beliefs were being translated into "science," and the ovaries and uterus were considered to be the ultimate controlling organs in woman, influencing not only her physical but also her psychological well-being. Since the ovaries and uterus controlled a woman's personality, eliminating these organs was viewed as a logical cure for psychological problems—thus, castration became a popular form of psychiatric treatment. Even tuberculosis, which took the lives of many young women, was believed to originate in the reproductive organs. Women were viewed as frail and susceptible to illness, and they were encouraged to be invalids. This cult of invalidism, however, was reserved for women of the middle- and upper classes; working-class women were allowed the day off to deliver their babies—a striking example of the impact of cultural, economic, and political systems on the treatment and behavior of women (Ehrenreich & English, 1973).

Today, we know that tuberculosis is caused by bacteria and that removing the ovaries does not cure psychological problems. On the other hand, the view of women as biologically determined has continued to be prevalent during our society: the primary roles available to women have been those related to reproduction; and the elderly woman has been viewed not as a valuable member of society because of her wisdom and experience but as devalued because of her loss of youthful beauty and fertility.

Popular views of a woman's reproductive life might be described as "Catch-22." According to cultural stereotypes, the week preceding menstruation is characterized by depression and irritability, and menstruation is accompanied by pain and discomfort, suggesting that women are incapacitated approximately half of the time. Given such attitudes, menopause should be welcomed as an end to such difficulties; however, cultural attitudes do not necessarily obey the rules of logic, and menopause is also viewed as a negative state associated with a host of physical and psychological problems. In a similarly paradoxical vein, women's psychology and behavior have been traditionally and inextricably linked to their biology—the hormonal pattern of the premenstruum renders women unbalanced, the physiological state of pregnancy is associated with uncharacteristic behaviors and whims. Nevertheless, any disordering of these processes—dysmenorrhea, excessively painful childbirth—are said to be caused not by biological disturbances, but by psychological ones.

Premenstrual syndrome and dysmenorrhea have traditionally been viewed as psychological problems; women complaining of either were seen as neurotic or as rejecting femininity. This perspective, combined with an attitude toward women as natural invalids whose illnesses did not matter because they did not hold valued positions, created a milieu that was not particularly conducive for the healing professions to develop verifiable theories that would logically lead to effective treatments. Menopause, on the other hand, has been considered a medical disorder, and the accompanying reduction in estrogen levels was considered the source of all ills in women over 50—an orientation that ignored the potential impact of stress and negative self-perceptions due to our cultural devaluation of the elderly. The recent women's movement is helping to change such theoretical orientations and, ultimately, to change the direction and emphasis of scholarly work. Not only are women demanding to be useful and productive members of society, but they are also insisting on safe contraception and effective treatments for dysmenorrhea, premenstrual syndrome, and menopausal symptoms in order to control their own reproduction and daily lives. Such demands, thus far, have been met with varying degrees of success.

Changing perspectives on and by women are also causing questions to be raised concerning the role of scientists in perpetuating the myth of women's inferiority. For example, consider the research on estrogen treatment for menopausal symptoms. It is fairly well established that estrogen is effective in relieving hot flashes and, perhaps, atrophic vaginitis, but it is not an effective treatment for other symptoms. It is also known that estrogen treatment is associated with an increased risk of uterine cancer. Thus, one would expect that a major goal of researchers would be to determine the minimum dose of estrogen effective in relieving hot flashes. Instead, research in this area has been designed from the perspective that hot flashes are not the problem but only a symptom of the problem, and the problem is menopause itself. Consequently, the vast majority of studies have sought to determine the dose of estrogen necessary to restore premenopausal hormonal values; as these doses are generally considerably higher than those required to relieve hot flashes, women are given estrogen in unnecessary and potentially dangerous quantities.

According to early theories of disease, biological and psychological symptoms were caused by biological and psychological factors, respectively, with psychosomatic disorders viewed as involving both etiological realms. We now know that psychological stress can increase one's vulnerability to colds and cancer and that biological disorders can influence one's vulnerability to depression. The controversy between psychiatry and psychology as to whether depression is due to central neurotransmitter depletion or to environmental stress has become meaningless with findings indicating that environmental stress can cause neurotransmitter depletion. Biological researchers are acknowledging the forces of culture and psychological processes on disease, and psychologists are hypothesizing biological predispositions in the development of psychological disorders. Thus, theories of the various disciplines are merging, primarily because the explanatory power of any one discipline is inadequate and unimpressive; it is time for a similar merging of the theories and research concerned with menstrual disorders and menopausal symptoms.

The purpose of this book is to present an integration and synthesis of scholarly work on the biological, psychological, and cultural aspects of menstruation, menstrual disorders, and menopause. The need for such a work has been brought about by a variety of recent advances that have broad implications across disciplines and are most productively interpreted within an integrative context. For example, it has become clear that dysmenorrhea is accompanied by elevated prostaglandins, substances that promote painful muscular activity, and drugs that inhibit the release of prostaglandins are effective during the treatment of dysmenorrhea for most women. However, such findings do not negate the fact that attitudes, expectations, beliefs, moods, and environmental stressors are associated with physiological patterns that have a potential effect on a woman's biological vulnerability to dysmenorrhea. Similarly, women who have interesting careers, who are physically and intellectually active, and who concentrate on the positive rather than the negative aspects of menopause tend to complain of fewer menopausal symptoms. Concluding from this that menopausal symptoms are exclusively a psychological reaction to old age and the loss of fertility is just as limiting and inadequate as attributing all such symptoms to estrogen deficiency.

In conclusion, my goal during writing this book was not to resolve the controversy regarding biological versus psychological causation but to discuss the mutually interacting and additive effects of biological, psychological, and cultural variables that influence the predisposition, development, maintenance, and treatment of menstrual disorders and menopausal symptoms.

I

THE HUMAN
MENSTRUAL CYCLE

1

Neuroendocrinological Aspects of the Menstrual Cycle

Overview

The reproductive cycle in woman is characterized by regular and predictable changes in endocrinological, physiological, and physical processes. It has an average periodicity of 28 days. The cycle begins in the ovary with the development of a follicle containing an immature egg. At maturation, ovulation occurs and the egg or ovum is released, and the corpus luteum develops from the remaining follicle. The ovum descends within the oviduct while the lining of the uterus proliferates in preparation for the fertilized ovum. If fertilization occurs, the embryo implants in the lining of the uterus to develop into a fetus. In the absence of fertilization, the ovum and the corpus luteum disintegrate, and the uterine lining is shed, resulting in menstruation. Toward the end of menstruation, follicular development begins once again and a new cycle commences.

These events, which characterize normal menstrual function, rely primarily on the activities of the hypothalamus, the anterior pituitary, and the ovaries. Beginning with menstruation as an arbitrary starting point, the hypothalamus produces gonadotropin-releasing hormone, which, in turn, stimulates the anterior pituitary to release the gonadotropins—follicle-stimulating hormone and luteinizing hormone. Follicle-stimulating hormone triggers the initial growth of follicles in the ovary. As these follicles develop, they begin to produce estrogen; eventually, one follicle assumes dominance and continues to develop, while the others regress. The domi-

3

∴ the pill + pregnancy

nant follicle increases its production of estrogen, and one action of this hormone is to cause proliferation of the endometrium, the lining of the uterus. Estrogen from the follicle also exerts a feedback effect on the anterior pituitary and is responsible for the midcycle surge of luteinizing hormone. This surge is followed by ovulation, which is the release of the mature ovum from the follicle. Luteinizing hormone also acts to transform the ruptured follicle into the corpus luteum. This preovulatory phase is referred to as the follicular or proliferative phase and is variable in length, typically ranging from 10 to 17 days.

In the postovulatory phase, the corpus luteum, a short-lived secretory organ, produces estrogen and progesterone. Progesterone acts to transform the endometrium into a secretory organ in preparation for implantation of the embryo if conception should occur. It also exerts a negative feedback effect on the release of gonadotropins from the pituitary, precluding further follicular growth during this phase. If conception does not occur, the corpus luteum degenerates, accompanied by decreasing levels of estrogen and progesterone. Since the secretory endometrium requires these hormones for maintenance, it also regresses, and menstruation occurs. Without the further inhibitory action of estrogen and progesterone, the anterior pituitary once again begins releasing gonadotropins, and a new cycle begins. This postovulatory phase is referred to as the luteal or secretory phase, and its duration of 13 to 15 days is relatively constant.

Regulatory Mechanisms

The hypothalamus secretes specific neurohormonal releasing factors which stimulate the synthesis and/or release of a variety of hormones from the pituitary. The releasing hormone most relevant to the menstrual cycle is gonadotropin-releasing hormone (GnRH), which stimulates the release of follicle-stimulating hormone (FSH) and luteinizing hormone (LH) from the anterior pituitary. Interestingly, FSH and LH release are not highly correlated in the menstrual cycle, and although this can be explained in a variety of ways, such as interactions with the concentrations of other hormones, some have argued that this lack of covariation between LH and FSH indicates that there may be two hypothalamic-releasing hormones, one targeted for LH, the other for FSH (Schally, Arimura, & Kastin, 1973). In the absence of any concrete evidence, however, one releasing hormone (GnRH) will be assumed to be responsible for the

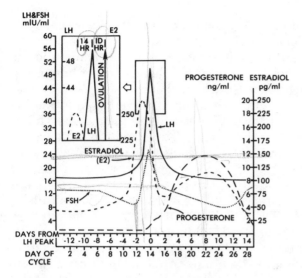

Figure 1.1. The temporal relationship of gonadotropin and ovarian steroid secretion in the normal menstrual cycle.

From M. A. Fritz and L. Speroff, The endocrinology of the menstrual cycle: The interaction of folliculogenesis and neuroendocrine mechanisms. *Fertility and Sterility, 38*:409, 1982. Reproduced with permission of the publisher, The American Fertility Society.

release of both gonadotropins in the present discussion. (Figure 1.1 graphically depicts the hormonal changes that occur during the menstrual cycle.)

It is believed that neurotransmitters of the catecholamine family may modulate the release of GnRH (Fritz & Speroff, 1983). Moreover, it has been hypothesized that GnRH secretion is regulated by a dual catecholaminergic system in which dopamine is inhibitory and norepinephrine is facilitory, and midcycle LH changes have been found to be associated with similar changes in urinary and plasma norepinephrine levels (Badano et al., 1978; Zuspan & Zuspan, 1973). Zuspan and Zuspan (1973) have concluded that progesterone and estrogen act in a synergistic fashion to modulate levels of norepinephrine, which, in turn, alter the pattern of GnRH release. Reviewing the research on the changes in LH produced by administration of dopamine and dopamine agonists, Yen (1980) has suggested that dopamine has a direct inhibitory effect on GnRH release. Research substantiating these neurotransmitter roles in the release of GnRH is continuing, but the majority of available research does support these hypotheses. Furthermore, as will become clear throughout this discussion of the menstrual cycle, physical, hormonal, and neurotransmitter changes that occur in the menstrual cycle interact in an extremely complex manner, so that, for example, the specific effects of a particular hormone may be dependent on the concentrations and previous patterns of release of other hormones.

The mode of action of GnRH on the anterior pituitary was initially thought to be neural, but direct innervation from the hypothalamus to the anterior pituitary was found to be absent. It has since been discovered that the hypothalamus and the pituitary are linked by a portal venous network such that virtually all of the blood flowing into the pituitary comes from the hypothalamus and will, thus, carry to the pituitary any hypothalamic hormone that has been released. In this manner GnRH reaches the anterior pituitary, and the presence of GnRH in the blood that profuses the pituitary causes the release of LH and FSH (Krieger, 1980).

GnRH is produced by the hypothalamus in a pulsatile rather than a steady fashion, and alterations in the amount of GnRH released are presumably reflected in changes in the quantity of LH and FSH released by the anterior pituitary. As discussed earlier, the gonadal steroids, estrogen and progesterone, play a role in regulating the amount of LH and FSH released by modulating the magnitude and frequency of GnRH secretion; however, there is strong evidence that estrogen and progesterone exert greater effects on LH and FSH release through a direct action on the anterior pituitary than by an indirect action on GnRH released from the hypothalamus. Indeed, Aksel (1979) measured plasma concentrations of GnRH in daily samples of normally ovulating women and noted that the mean GnRH level coincident with the LH midcycle surge is not significantly different from the mean follicular or luteal phase concentrations. In a later report, Aksel (1981) found GnRH and LH levels to be significantly correlated only in early follicular days, and no relation was found between GnRH concentrations and FSH release in any cycle day. These data suggest that the cyclic pattern exhibited by LH and FSH is not primarily due to a similar cyclic pattern of GnRH release, that estrogen and progesterone influence the synthesis and/or release of the gonadotropins, and that the target of the feedback is apparently the pituitary rather than the hypothalamus. Fritz and Speroff (1983) suggest that GnRH is necessary but not sufficient in the control of gonadotropin secretion and that the feedback of the gonadal steroids on the pituitary is largely responsible for the pattern of LH and FSH secretion observed in the menstrual cycle.

The manner in which the gonadal steroids affect gonadotropin release is complex. Two pools of gonadotropins have been hypothesized (Yen, 1980)—a reserve pool and a releasable pool, which together make up total pituitary capacity. In the early follicular phase both pools are at a minimum, and during the follicular phase the reserve pool increases preferentially; however, prior to mid-cycle, the pattern reverses, and releasable exceeds reserve. Both are high during the luteal phase, and then they decline. The reserve pool is the result of the priming effect of GnRH on pituitary capacity. This pool is augmented by a self-priming action of GnRH, in which GnRH receptors in the anterior pituitary increase in response to low but continuous exposure to GnRH (Hoff, Lasley, & Yen, 1979). In addition, high levels of estrogen facilitate this priming effect and further increase the size of the reserve pool. During the midfollicular phase of the menstrual cycle, the reserve pool increases with increasing levels of estrogen. Thus, pituitary responsiveness to GnRH is dependent on the duration of continuous GnRH levels and on the duration and concentration of circulating estrogen. These priming effects of GnRH and estrogen are reflected in a greater GnRH receptor concentration in the anterior pituitary and in a greater reserve pool of gonadotropins. This build-up of pituitary reserve is necessary to provide sufficient LH for the midcycle surge.

The second pool represents the releasable portion of pituitary capacity and reflects pituitary sensitivity to GnRH. During the late follicular and midcycle phases of the menstrual cycle, this pool increases preferentially in size. In contrast to the positive feedback effect of estrogen on the reserve pool, estrogen exerts negative feedback on the releasable pool; there is, however, lack of agreement as to whether this effect is mediated via the hypothalamus or the pituitary or both. Thus, it is hypothesized that estrogen stimulates the reserve pool but blocks the acute release of the gonadotropins.

Despite the crucial role that estrogen and progesterone play in regulating events associated with the menstrual cycle, there is some confusion as to the actual source of these steroids. Both hormones are produced by the ovaries, by the corpus luteum, and by the adrenal cortex, but it is difficult to determine the relative contribution of each of these sources. This is because progesterone may be converted to androstenedione, which, in turn, may be converted to estrogen; these conversions may take place prior to release by the various organs, or they may take place in peripheral tissue. A second difficulty in determining the source of these hormones relates to the fact that the term "estrogen" is a generic term for three substances, estradiol, estrone, and estriol, estradiol being the most biologically active form of the three. In general, it is believed that most circulating estradiol is produced by the follicle and the corpus luteum, while the majority of progesterone is produced by the corpus luteum. However, small amounts of both steroids are produced by the adrenal cortex or derived from peripheral conversion.

The Follicular Phase and Ovulation

The primary activity of the preovulatory phase of the menstrual cycle is the selection and subsequent development of the dominant follicle. Although the stimulus for the initiation of follicular growth is unclear, progressive development is dependent upon the interaction between the gonadotropins and the ovarian steroids. Once growth has begun, the follicle is capable of synthesizing estrogen, progesterone, and androgens; estrogen, however, is the primary hormone secreted (Fritz & Speroff, 1983). FSH, secreted by the anterior pituitary, is self-enhancing in that it tends to raise the concentration of its own receptor: FSH in concert with estrogen acts to facilitate follicular growth, and, as the follicle increases in size, its capacity for estrogen production is enhanced (Kerin et al., 1981; Sanyal et al., 1974).

FSH and estrogen act synergistically to induce LH receptor development on the follicle. FSH and LH stimulate the ovarian production of androgens, which are then converted to estrogen through FSH-initiated aromatization. When the follicle attains sufficient size, estrogen production reaches magnitudes that produce feedback effects on gonadotropin production. Estrogen enhances the actions of FSH within the follicle but inhibits FSH and LH release at the hypothalamic–pituitary level. Fritz and Speroff (1983) have suggested that this dual action of estrogen may ensure that only one follicle develops—the one with the largest production of estrogen—while others fail due to decreasing levels of FSH.

Other factors may also contribute to the selection of a single dominant follicle. The dominant follicle produces a substance referred to as "inhibin," which has negative feedback effects on pituitary production of FSH (Fritz & Speroff, 1983). In addition, a protein that is secreted by the ovary containing the dominant follicle, which suppresses the gonadotropin responsivity of other follicles of its own as well as the contralateral ovary, has been identified (DiZerega, Goebelsmann, & Nakamura, 1982).

The end result of the opposing effects of estrogen on the two pools of gonadotropins is an augmentation of pituitary capacity, which builds steadily during middle and late follicular phases in synchrony with rising levels of estrogen (Cutler & Garcia, 1980). This build-up culminates in the midcycle surges of LH and FSH. Disagreement exists as to the trigger for the gonadotropin surge. Some researchers have suggested that the trigger might be a particular level of circulating estrogen or possibly a particular rate of increase of estrogen (Hoff, Quigley, & Yen, 1983; March et al., 1979). However, there is a lack of consensus as to the required level and duration of estrogen; Fritz and Speroff (1983) have stated that 200 pg/ml (picograms per milliliter) of estrogen maintained for 50 hours is required for the LH surge, whereas Yen (1980) has suggested 300 pg/ml for 72 hours.

In contrast, data from several reports (Moghissi, Syner, & Evans, 1972; World Health Organization, 1981) indicate that both serum and urinary levels of estradiol peak and then start to decline at least one day prior to the LH surge, suggesting that falling levels of estrogen may be the trigger. The latter explanation more logically fits with the previously stated theory that estrogen blocks release of the gonadotropins, since falling estrogen levels would then decrease the estrogen-induced inhibition. However, some empirical evidence does not particularly favor either theory, as exemplified by one study (Thorneycroft et al., 1974) that found that serum estradiol levels had started to decline in two subjects, but not in a third, prior to the LH surge.

Although the role of progesterone in the midcycle gonadotropin surge has not been researched as thoroughly as that of estrogen, progesterone does apparently contribute and may, in fact, be necessary to the normal sequence of events leading to ovulation. Toward the end of follicular growth, luteinization of the follicle begins; specialized cells become hypertrophied and begin to secrete progesterone (Thorneycroft et al., 1971). Although the source of progesterone later in the cycle is the corpus luteum, this steroid can be detected in the blood 24 to 48 hours prior to ovulation and the development of the corpus luteum, and thus it has been assumed that the source of this early progesterone is the follicle (Fritz & Speroff, 1983).

Several investigators (Hoff, Quigley, & Yen, 1983; World Health Organization, 1981) have reported a rise in progesterone approximately 12 hours prior to the onset of the surge in LH, a finding that is consistent with the fact that small amounts of progesterone are known to augment GnRH-mediated LH release. March and colleagues, (1979) administered estrogen and progesterone to oophorectomized women of reproductive age. Infusions mimicking the preovulatory estradiol peak were followed by an LH surge but not one of FSH. However, when progesterone was added after estradiol, the LH surge was accompanied by an FSH peak. The authors conclude that both estrogen and progesterone levels are crucial in effecting typical midcycle gonadotropin surges. Approximately 18 hours after FSH and LH peak, the mature follicle ruptures, and ovulation occurs.

The Luteal Phase and Menstruation

The time between ovulation and menstruation is variously referred to as the postovulatory, luteal, or secretory phase. The first event to occur during this phase is the formation of the corpus luteum. The corpus luteum is a secretory structure on the surface of the ovary that develops within the ruptured ovarian follicle. It is essentially a short-lived endocrine organ and secretes both progesterone and estrogen. The life span and capacity of the corpus luteum to produce estrogen and progesterone are dependent upon the continued release of LH from the pituitary (Fritz & Speroff, 1983). On the other hand, the steroids secreted by the corpus luteum exert negative feedback effects on the release of the gonadotropins (Taymor & Thompson, 1975). New follicular growth is inhibited, not only by the lowered levels of the gonadotropins, but also by progesterone, which acts directly on the ovary to inhibit new follicular growth during the luteal phase.

If fertilization of the ovum does not occur, the corpus luteum gradually decreases production of progesterone and estrogen, and it eventually atrophies prior to menstruation. Although the cause of luteal regression or luteolysis is unknown, several hypotheses have been suggested. For example, Bolton, Coulam, and Ryan (1980) noted that the number of LH receptors in the corpus luteum decreases gradually, which could well explain decreased steroidogenesis and loss of sensitivity to LH, but they do not speculate as to the nature of the mechanism that causes the decrease in LH receptor concentration.

Prostaglandins have been proposed as a possible luteolytic agent. Prostaglandins are unsaturated fatty acids that have actions similar to hormones, but they are synthesized in tissues other than glands. Originally discovered in human seminal fluid, they have since been found to be concentrated in the lung, kidney, and uterus and are typically released by such mechanical stimuli as stretching, squeezing, and compression (Fuchs, 1977). Certain prostaglandins—those in groups E and F—covary with the menstrual cycle. The two main smooth-muscle-stimulating prostaglandins, PGE_2 and PGF_{2a}, are found in the endometrium and menstrual fluid (Speroff & Ramwell, 1970). Endometrial content of these prostaglandins is low during proliferative and early luteal phases. As the cycle progresses, PGF_{2a} increases continually from early luteal through late luteal phases to menstruation, while PGE_2 remains low until the late luteal phase, when it increases until menstruation (Maathius, 1978; Singh, Baccarini, & Zuspan, 1975; Willman, Collins, & Clayton, 1976). Plasma levels of prostaglandins have also been reported to fluctuate in a similar manner: Van Orden and associates (1977) found that while plasma PGF_{2a} did not exhibit significant variation during the menstrual cycle, PGE_2 did vary significantly, with the low point approximately 8 days prior to the LH surge and the high point 16 days after it.

With regard to corpus luteum regression, Cutler and Carcia (1980) have suggested that prostaglandins, in conjunction with estrogen, are responsible for luteolysis. According to their theory, estrogen, produced by the corpus luteum, acts to effect changes in the endometrium, which, in turn, synthesizes and releases prostaglandins, which then contribute to the regression of the corpus luteum. However, Aksel, Schomberg, and Hammond (1977) reported that the higher concentrations of PGF_{2a} seen in the luteal phases were not accompanied by a decrease in progesterone, which one would expect if this prostaglandin were influential in initiating luteolysis. Additionally, Fritz and Speroff (1983) have reviewed evidence suggesting that exogenous estrogen induces luteolysis, and that this estrogen-induced luteolysis can be blocked by inhibiting prostaglandin synthesis. Furthermore, prostaglandin receptors have been found in the plasma membrane of the human corpus luteum (Arrata & Tsai, 1978). Thus, physiologically, it appears possible that estrogen and prostaglandins may act in conjunction to initiate luteolysis, but it remains to be proven that this process occurs in the normal menstrual cycle.

Prostaglandins have also been implicated in events immediately preceding and accompanying menstruation. Jordan and Pokoly (1977) measured estrogen and progesterone levels in peripheral and uterine venous plasma and PGF and PGE levels in peripheral and uterine venous plasma and in endometrial curettage samples at various phases of the menstrual cycle. While uterine PGF content was directly related to estradiol levels in the uterine venous plasma, the highest concentration of PGF was found during the secretory phase in the presence of progesterone. The authors interpreted their data as suggesting that low levels of progesterone are necessary for estradiol to stimulate PGF synthesis, but that higher levels of progesterone, as occur during the midluteal phase, may suppress the release of prostaglandins, resulting in the accumulation of prostaglandins in endometrial cells. When progesterone levels fall abruptly, as they do in the late luteal phase, the high concentrations of stored PGF might be released, causing a variety of events that accompany menstruation such as tissue breakdown and uterine contractions.

The Endometrium

Throughout the menstrual cycle, changes occur in the endometrium. The endometrium is the mucous membrane lining of the uterus and consists of the stratum compactum, the stratum spongiosum, and the stratum basale—the former two being the layers shed during menstruation. After menstruation, only a thin layer of basal cells remain. The estrogen secreted by the developing follicle acts on the endometrium and causes the cells in the two surface strata to proliferate rapidly. The endometrium is resurfaced within 3 to 7 days after the beginning of menstruation. During the remaining portion of the preovulatory phase, increasing levels of estrogen cause the endometrium to increase 5- to 10-fold in thickness, due to an increasing number of stromal cells and the growth of endometrial glands and the blood vessels required to supply the endometrium.

After ovulation, estrogen and progesterone are secreted by the corpus luteum, causing further cellular proliferation, and the thickness approximately doubles during this phase. The progesterone causes the endometrium to convert to a secretory stage—that is, the cells change to mucus-producing glands. Some cells begin to store nutrients in preparation for pregnancy, and vascularization increases. If fertilization does not occur, then progesterone production, which maintains the secretory endometrium, begins to decline. This results in involution of the endometrium, and the blood vessels become vasospastic. This, in turn, leads to endometrial necrosis, shedding of the necrotic layers, and, eventually, menstruation, which is the expulsion of the desquamated tissue and blood.

In order for progesterone to exert its effects during the secretory phase of the menstrual cycle, the endometrium must first be stimulated by estrogen. During the preovulatory phase, estrogen increases the endometrial response to itself by causing an increase in the concentration of its own receptor; interestingly, estrogen also increases the concentration of progesterone receptors (Natrajan et al., 1981). The concentration of progesterone receptors in the endometrium is at a maximum at the time of ovulation—at the precise time that progesterone begins to be secreted (Schmidt-Gollwitzer et al., 1979). One action of progesterone during the secretory phase is to cause a decrease in estrogen receptor concentration, while a second is to increase the conversion rate of estradiol to a less potent estrogen, estrone (Jacobs, Suchocki, & Smith, 1980). The resulting decrease in estrogenic activity, in turn, probably diminishes the stimulation of progesterone receptors by estrogen, resulting in a nadir of steroid receptor concentration in the endometrium in the late secretory phase (Levy et al., 1980).

Summary

Selection and development of a dominant follicle, ovulation, corpus luteum maintenance, and cyclic changes in the endometrium are all necessary in maintaining reproductive potential. These processes depend upon a precise coordination and a delicate balance of hypothalamic-pituitary secretions and ovarian steroidogenesis. Research during the last decade has not only significantly contributed to our understanding of the menstrual cycle, but also provided an appreciation of the tremendous complexity that characterizes the regulation of this cycle: the steroid production of the corpus luteum depends upon continued release of LH, but the steroids produced exert negative feedback on the pituitary, which inhibits release of LH; during the preovulatory phase, estrogen acts to enhance the effect of FSH within the follicle but inhibits FSH release at the hypothalamic-pituitary level; follicular development and ovulation are directly dependent upon concentrations of gonadotropins, which, in turn, are influenced by estrogen, progesterone, norepinephrine, and GnRH and their interactive effects. Although there has been considerable progress in recent years in terms of delineating the subtleties of these interacting systems, a variety of mechanisms—such as the stimulus for initiation of follicular growth, the trigger for the gonadotropin surge immediately preceding ovulation, and the cause of luteolysis—remain a mystery.

Although past research has concentrated on the ovary as the initiator and regulator of normal cyclic functioning, the current emphasis is on the brain as the ultimate controller of interactions among the hypothalamus, anterior pituitary, and ovaries. Thus, alterations in central nervous system activity resulting from environmental events or psychological stress may influence menstrual cycle functioning, and, conversely, alterations in hormonal levels may influence mood. Furthermore, the neuroendocrinological patterns associated with the menstrual cycle impact to various degrees on almost every physiological system in the body, and, conversely, a host of exogenous and endogenous factors may alter or interfere with the normal menstrual cycle.

2

Central Nervous System Activity Associated with the Menstrual Cycle

As shown in the preceding chapter, regulation of the menstrual cycle is extremely complex. The positive and negative feedback systems among releasing hormones, gonadotropins, and ovarian steroids maintain a continually changing, but precisely controlled, internal milieu. These interactive systems affect every physiological system in the body and are, in turn, affected by a wide variety of internal and external events. Given that environmental stimuli, psychological stress, and belief systems impact on the menstrual cycle, the ultimate integration of internal and external influences must necessarily be in the central nervous sytem. Thus, normal menstrual cycle regulation is dependent upon the biochemical actions of the central nervous system, particularly the activity of neurotransmitters.

Catecholamines

Two neurotransmitters, important in regulating the menstrual cycle, are dopamine and norepinephrine—neurotransmitters that belong to the more general class of catecholamines. Catecholamines are formed in the brain and the sympathetic nervous system from the amino acid tyrosine. Tyrosine undergoes a series of chemical transformations, resulting in the formation of dopamine, norepine-phrine, or epinephrine. Tyrosine is found in many foods, and it is

15

also derived from dietary phenylalanine, which can be converted to tyrosine by the enzyme phenylalanine hydroxylase, found primarily in the liver. Tyrosine is then converted to dihydroxyphenylalanine (DOPA) through the actions of the enzyme tyrosine hydroxylase. The activity of tyrosine hydroxylase is inhibited by increased levels of catecholamines, suggesting that dopamine and norepinephrine may control their own rates of synthesis by exerting negative feedback inhibition on the formation of tyrosine hydroxylase. Therefore, the conversion of tyrosine to DOPA is the rate-limiting step in the synthesis of catecholamines.

A second enzyme, DOPA-decarboxylase, converts DOPA to dopamine. Dopamine is a neurotransmitter in its own right and, in addition, serves as a precursor for norepinephrine. Dopamine-beta-hydroxylase hydroxylizes dopamine to norepinephrine and is an inductible enzyme in that its activity can be increased by stress and by certain drugs such as reserpine. Phenylethanolamine-N-Methyl transferase causes the enzymatic conversion of norepinephrine to epinephrine in the adrenal glands.

Dopamine and norepinephrine perform their neurotransmitter function by being released from axon terminals into synaptic clefts and then by binding to specific receptors on postsynaptic cells. Their actions are terminated principally by reuptake of the neurotransmitters back into the presynaptic nerve terminals, where they are reincorporated into vesicles for subsequent release or metabolized by monoamine oxidase. Some catecholamines are also metabolized at postsynaptic cells through the actions of another enzyme known as catechol-O-methyltransferase (COMT).

An obvious and noninvasive method for studying the interactions among hormones, gonadotropins, and neurotransmitters is to assess the concentrations of catecholamines at different points in time during the normal menstrual cycle. Such investigations have yielded few meaningful results. Zacur and colleagues (1978) obtained plasma samples regularly throughout the menstrual cycle in 6 normally menstruating women. They analyzed the plasma for LH, FSH, prolactin, norepinephrine, and dopamine-beta-hydroxylase (DBH)—the latter being the enzyme that mediates the conversion of dopamine to norepinephrine. No consistent pattern of change was found in either DBH or norepinephrine concentrations during the cycle, and DBH and norepinephrine did not correlate significantly with either gonadotropin, nor with prolactin.

In contrast, Redmond and coworkers (1975) found significant cycle effects for DBH in rhesus monkeys with the peak around menses and the nadir at midcycle. Further, Weiner and Elmadjian

(1962) reported significantly greater urinary norepinephrine levels during the premenstruum than during the several days immediately after menses in a woman suffering from premenstrual tension. Unfortunately, the subject samples, the inconsistent results, and the lack of programmatic research preclude the drawing of any definitive conclusions as to the patterns of change in catecholamines throughout the cycle in normally menstruating women.

There appears to be greater consistency in those studies that have concentrated specifically on the biochemical events surrounding ovulation. Zuspan and Zuspan (1973) reported an increase in plasma norepinephrine and epinephrine at the approximate time of ovulation, although they did not find parallel changes in urinary catecholamines. Similar results were found by Rosner and coworkers (1976), who assessed plasma levels of norepinephrine, LH, and estradiol daily prior to and subsequent to ovulation in three normally ovulating women. Plasma norepinephrine began to rise rapidly one day prior to, or concomitant with, the LH peak. Injections of GnRH on Day 10 in four other subjects resulted in a similar rapid rise in plasma norepinephrine. In a third study (Badano et al., 1978) blood was sampled every eight hours around the expected time of ovulation; 8 hours after estradiol peaked and 48 hours prior to the LH surge, plasma norepinephrine concentrations increased, reaching a maximum 24 hours after the estradiol peak. Interpretations of these studies vary—Zuspan and Zuspan (1973) suggested that the release of norepinephrine from nerve stores triggers the release of GnRH, while Rosner and coworkers (1976) interpreted their data to mean that GnRH release results in a rise in norepinephrine levels.

A study using rats by Katra and McCann (1974), although not resolving this issue, does point out the necessary role of catecholamines in ovulation. Both inhibition of catecholamine synthesis with alpha methyl paratyrosine, a tyrosine hydroxylase inhibitor, and depletion of brain norepinephrine stores with diethyldithiocarbamate, a dopamine-beta-hydroxylase inhibitor, blocked both the preovulatory LH surge and ovulation in proestrous rats. They were unable to reverse this blockade by administering L-DOPA, a finding consistent with studies discussed below, which suggest that dopamine inhibits and norepinephrine facilitates gonadotropin release.

Several studies have investigated the effects of exogenously administered dopamine or L-DOPA, a precursor of dopamine, on the hypothalamic-pituitary system. Leblanc and colleagues (1976) found that an infusion of dopamine resulted in a significant reduction in LH, while Lachelin, Leblanc, and Yen (1977) noted a similar reduction in LH following administration of L-DOPA. Leebaw, Lee, and Woolf (1978) found basal LH levels in six men unaffected by dopamine infusion, but the LH response to exogenous GnRH was inhibited.

Other studies assessed the variation in effects of dopamine on LH as a function of the phase of the menstrual cycle. In women subjects, Judd, Rakoff, and Yen (1978) reported minimal inhibition of LH by dopamine during those phases of the menstrual cycle when basal levels of LH were low, but a dramatic inhibition when basal levels were high prior to ovulation; the correlation between basal LH and the magnitude of the response to dopamine was 0.979. Yen (1980) interpreted these results as implying that the mechanism of dopamine inhibition is due to a direct effect on GnRH release rather than on LH secretion from the anterior pituitary. However, a later study by Huseman, Kugler, and Schneider (1980) suggested that dopamine interferes with the action of GnRH after it is released. They administered dopamine and GnRH separately and together to male subjects. Dopamine alone suppressed the frequency and amplitude of LH pulsatile release, while GnRH increased LH release. However, this effect of GnRH was significantly suppressed when dopamine was administered together with GnRH.

Neurotransmitter–hormonal interactions are further complicated when the potential mediating role of estrogen is considered. Judd, Rigg, and Yen (1979) compared the suppressive action of dopamine on LH release in ovariectomized and normal women. Consistent with previous studies that noted greater suppression at higher basal levels of LH, the suppressive effect was greater in the ovariectomized women who had high basal levels of LH. Furthermore, they found that pretreatment with estrogen lowered basal LH levels and thereby proportionately decreased the suppressive effects of dopamine. Estrogen, however, appears to affect dopamine-induced suppression of LH by lowering basal LH levels rather than through any direct action on the metabolism of dopamine, since Judd, Rakoff, and Yen (1978) found that the degree of dopamine suppression varied with basal LH levels but not with basal estrogen levels during the normal cycle.

On the other hand, evidence from studies assessing changes in catecholamines following ovariectomy suggests that estrogen does, indeed, affect concentrations of circulating catecholamines. Anton-Tay and Wurtman (1968) found an increase in plasma norepinephrine following ovariectomy. In a later study, LaTorre (1974) reported that ovariectomy in the rat resulted in increased central norepinephrine levels and decreased central dopamine levels; furthermore, estradiol replacement reversed these trends, increasing dopamine and decreasing norepinephrine. Such research recently led several theorists in the area (Coulam, 1981; Fritz & Speroff, 1983) to conclude that reductions in estrogen, including reductions brought about by ovariectomy, result in increased norepinephrine and decreased dopamine, while the administration of estrogen has the opposite effect. Janowsky and Davis (1970), in a perhaps overly enthusiastic interpretation of these data, suggest that estrogen and progesterone be classified along with reserpine, monoamine oxidase inhibitors, and tricyclics as pharmacological agents that affect mood states.

Prolactin, a hormone secreted by the anterior pituitary, also covaries with catecholamines. Fairly consistent findings indicate that prolactin levels in the blood decrease in response to increased dopamine (Langer & Sachar, 1977; Leblanc et al., 1976), the dopamine precursor L-DOPA (Lacheline, Leblanc, & Yen, 1977; Leblanc & Yen, 1976), and the dopamine agonist methyldopa (Steiner et al., 1976). Other studies support such a relationship by indicating that drugs that attenuate the effects of dopamine increase plasma prolactin levels. Thus, prolactin has been demonstrated to increase in response to phenothiazines—dopamine receptor antagonists—(Buckman & Peake, 1973; Leblanc & Yen, 1976; Tolis, Dent, & Guyda, 1978; Tyson & Friesen, 1973), other neuroleptics (Langer & Sachar, 1977), as well as morphine and methadone (Tolis, Dent, & Guyda, 1978). Langer and coworkers (1977b) observed dose–response relationships between several types of phenothiazines and plasma prolactin levels. In a second study (Langer et al., 1977a), this same research group found a highly significant correlation between prolactin release effectiveness and antischizophrenic potency in a variety of drugs at various dosages. Furthermore, Leblanc and Yen (1976) found that L-DOPA induced decreases in prolactin followed by a rebound increase and that the amount of suppression was similar to that of rebound; they concluded that dopamine blocked secretion, but not synthesis, of prolactin.

Buckman, Peake, and Srivastava (1976) found that endogenous levels of estrogen modulated phenothiazine-stimulated prolactin secretion. They measured the prolactin response to phenothiazines in the early follicular phase, when estrogen levels are low, and compared this value to the response in the late follicular phase, when estrogen levels are higher. Although mean serum prolactin levels were similar in each phase of the cycle, the magnitude of the prolactin response to the phenothiazine was significantly greater when estrogen levels were high than when they were low, suggesting that estrogen may affect prolactin production; the authors did not speculate about the exact mechanism involved.

Judd and colleagues (Judd, Rakoff, & Yen, 1978; Judd, Rigg, & Yen, 1979) investigated the effects of endogenous and exogenously administered estrogen as well as basal prolactin levels on the inhibiting effects of dopamine on prolactin release. In their earlier study, the inhibition of prolactin release by dopamine correlated well with plasma estrogen concentrations ($r = .685$) and also with basal prolactin levels ($r = .878$). In the latter study, the inhibition of prolactin release by dopamine was less in ovariectomized women than in normal women, and the degree of inhibition was increased if dopamine administration was preceded by exogenous estrogen.

One possible physiological mechanism responsible for these prolactin–neurotransmitter interactions has been described by Fournier, Desjardins, and Friesen (1974). They suggested that prolactin secretion is controlled primarily by prolactin-inhibiting factor (PIF) released from the hypothalamus and transported in the portal capillary system to the anterior pituitary. The rate of secretion of PIF is controlled by a hypothalamic catecholamine, probably dopamine. Conditions or experimental treatments that deplete catecholamines cause a decrease in PIF, leading to an increase in prolactin release, while conditions that enhance catecholamine levels have the opposite effect.

Serotonin

Serotonin, another important neurotransmitter, is synthesized in the brain and other parts of the body from tryptophan—an amino acid derived primarily from the diet. The rate-limiting step in the synthesis of serotonin is the hydroxylation of tryptophan to 5-hydroxytryptophan, a reaction catalyzed by the enzyme tryptophan hydroxylase. Then, serotonin is formed from 5-hydroxytryptophan through the action of 5-hydroxytryptophan decarboxylase. As a neurotransmitter, serotonin operates similarly to dopamine and norepinephrine; it is metabolized primarily by monoamine oxidase.

Serotonin and its metabolic precursor, tryptophan, have also been studied with respect to the menstrual cycle and their interactions with various hormones. In contrast to those effects of norepinephrine and dopamine on hormone release discussed above, alterations in serotonin systems, either decreased by a serotonergic receptor blocker (Kapen, Vagenakis, & Braverman, 1980) or increased by the administration of L-tryptophan, had little effect on plasma LH, FSH, or prolactin concentrations.

There is some evidence suggesting that ovarian hormones influence serotonin activity. Wood and Coppen (1978) treated depressed patients with estrogen and noted a significant increase in the level of free tryptophan. They concluded, however, that this was probably the result of a direct effect, since, in vitro, estrogen displaces tryptophan from plasma protein binding sites. Estrogen has also been shown to increase the rate of excretion of tryptophan metabolites (Coulam, 1981), and this excretion rate returned to normal with large doses of pyridoxine (vitamin B6) (Rose, 1972).

Consistent with these results are those reported in studies concerned with the effects of oral contraceptives on tryptophan metabolism. Price, Thornton, and Mueller (1967) assessed the excretion rate of xanthurenic acid, a tryptophan metabolite, in women ingesting oral contraceptives and in controls. The oral contraceptives had no significant effect on basal excretion, but a tryptophan-loading test resulted in the women using oral contraceptives excreting significantly more xanthurenic acid than did non-users. When vitamin B6 was administered to users, the excretion of tryptophan metabolites returned to normal. Increases in the excretion of tryptophan metabolites due to the ingestion of oral contraceptives and the correcting effect of pyridoxine has been a consistent finding in the literature (Rose & Adams, 1972; Rose et al., 1972). Others have found pyridoxine to relieve depression in women taking oral contraceptives (Adams et al., 1973; Baumblatt & Winston, 1970).

There has been some speculation as to the specific mechanisms involved in the relationships among oral contraceptives, tryptophan, and pyridoxine. The metabolism of tryptophan to tryptamine and serotonin is dependent on pyridoxine. If pyridoxine is insufficent, all tryptophan that has entered the metabolic cycle cannot be processed, and some will be excreted in the urine (Larsson-Cohn, 1975). Oral contraceptives may cause a lack of active pyridoxine by loosening the binding of some pyridoxine from its enzyme, which would result in inadequate decarboxylation of tryptophan and lower levels of serotonin (Winston, 1969). Adams and colleagues (1973) have suggested that the estrogen component in oral contraceptives is responsible for such an effect in that estrogen increases cortisol activity in the liver, and hydrocortisone administration greatly increases hepatic tryptophan oxygenase levels, which, in turn, increase the requirements of vitamin B6 to achieve normal production of serotonin.

Catecholestrogens

The accumulating evidence that estrogen exhibits central nervous system actions has stimulated interest in estrogen metabolism in the brain. Research has indicated that brain tissue, particularly the hypothalamus, is capable of conferring a catechol structure on the estrogen molecule, resulting in catecholestrogens. These compounds have the potential of interacting with both the catecholamine and the estrogen systems in the brain (Yen, 1980). Catechol-O-methyl transferase (COMT) metabolizes both catecholamines and catecholestrogens but exhibits a greater affinity for the latter. As a result, catecholestrogens can effectively compete for COMT and thus alter the metabolism of the neurotransmitters, which, in turn, may effect GnRH release and ultimately gonadotropin secretion (Fritz & Speroff, 1983). Yen (1980) has reported that catecholestrogens have the potential for inhibiting tyrosine hydroxylase, the rate-limiting enzyme involved in catecholamine synthesis. In this way, they may act to reduce neurotransmitter levels.

This is a relatively new area of research, but the available data suggest that catecholestrogens may mediate the feedback effects of estrogen on gonadotropin secretion. Schinfeld and colleagues (1980) administered catecholestrogens to postmenopausal women and compared those who had been pretreated with estrogen with those not pretreated. Without the estrogen prime, catecholestrogens had no consistent effect on LH, FSH, or prolactin concentrations. Those women who had received estrogen therapy, however, responded to catecholestrogens by exhibiting significant decreases in LH, FSH, and prolactin, although the LH decrease was preceded by an increase in the release of LH. Considerably more research is needed in order to further delineate the metabolism and actions of catecholestrogens and their interactions with other substances in the central nervous system. Research in this area, thus far, promises considerable potential for increasing our understanding of the biochemical regulation of the menstrual cycle.

Monoamine Oxidase

Of primary importance in the modulation of neurotransmitter function is monoamine oxidase (MAO), an enzyme associated with the mitochondria of neurons, which is responsible for the metabolism of dopamine, norepinephrine, and serotonin. MAO levels are inversely related to central adrenergic functioning, since MAO inactivates neural supplies of monoamines. Thus, conditions or experimental treatments that depress MAO concentrations are associated with increased levels of norepinephrine, dopamine, and serotonin.

Platelet MAO has been found to vary with the menstrual cycle in women (Belmaker et al., 1974) and in female rhesus monkeys (Redmond et al., 1975). In both, platelet MAO exhibited a preovulatory increase and a peak during midcycle. Gilmore and coworkers (1971) failed to find similar results but sampled blood only twice during the cycle. Others (Grant & Mears, 1967; Southgate et al., 1968) found endometrial MAP to vary with the cycle; both studies reported a significant increase in endometrial MAO in the late secretory phase.

Inconsistent findings have been reported concerning the variability in plasma MAO during the cycle. Redmond and colleagues (1975) and Gilmore and coworkers (1971) found no consistent pattern. In contrast, Klaiber and colleagues (1971) sampled blood more frequently than was done in other studies and found significantly more plasma MAO during the premenstrual week than during the preovulatory week. Integrating and interpreting such diverse results is difficult. Endometrial MAO fluctuations could well be a local rather than a systemic effect; and as platelet lifespan is about ten days, there could be a delay between changes in central MAO and detectable changes in platelet MAO. Most importantly, plasma, platelet, or endometrial MAO does not necessarily reflect central MAO activity.

On the other hand, an investigation by Vogel, Broverman, and Klaiber (1971) suggested that such variations in plasma MAO may, indeed, reflect central MAO activity. They studied the photic driving response of the electroencephalogram—a response that diminishes when central adrenergic functioning is enhanced—in normally menstruating and amenorrheic women treated with estrogen and estrogen plus progesterone. In the normally cycling women, there were fewer responses during the secretory phase than during the follicular phase; in the amenorrheic women, treatment with estrogen significantly reduced the driving response; and in most subjects, there were fewer responses with estrogen alone than with estrogen plus progesterone.

One reason for interest in the relationships between ovarian hormones and MAO is that increased levels of MAO have been shown to be associated with various states of depression (Klaiber et al., 1972), and, if MAO varies as a function of estrogen and/or progesterone levels, then premenstrual depression could, in theory, be due to changes in MAO resulting from hormonal changes. The increased levels of plasma MAO during the premenstruum are consistent with such a theory. Furthermore, Klaiber and colleagues (1971) found that exogenous estrogen resulted in a significant decrease in plasma MAO and that adding progesterone to the estrogen increased MAO levels above those produced by estrogen alone. Finally, menopausal women with lowered or absent estrogen synthesis have been found to have higher MAO activity than normally menstruating women (Englander-Golden, Willis, and Dienstbier, 1977). Although certainly not conclusive, these data imply that estrogen inhibits central MAO activity and that this inhibition, in turn, enhances adrenergic processes, while progesterone has the opposite effect.

Summary

The central nervous system and the pituitary-ovarian system are mutually interactive, and this reciprocity is manifest in the regulation and dysregulation of the menstrual cycle. However, caution should be exercised in drawing definitive conclusions, since research in this area is marked by considerable difficulties in methodology and interpretation; for example: (1) since hormonal effects depend upon binding with receptors, fluctuations in receptor concentrations can influence the biological impact of hormones without altering plasma levels; (2) when hormones are circulated in the plasma in a bound form, they are not biologically active, so that assays that measure total levels without differentiating bound from unbound forms are not necessarily indicative of the functional effects of the hormone (McClintock, 1981); (3) hormonal effects on the anterior pituitary and the central nervous system may depend upon whether the hormonal levels are normal or abnormal, on whether they are endogenous or altered with exogenous forms, on the levels of other substances such as binding globulins, on previous hormonal levels and rates of change, and, in the case of exogenously administered hormones, on whether the dose is a physiological or a pharmacological one.

Given these limitations and cautions, a few tentative conclusions can be drawn. Ovarian hormones have apparent effects on central nervous system activity; estrogen tends to increase dopamine concentrations but decrease concentrations of serotonin, norepinephrine, and MAO, while progesterone tends to increase MAO. In addition, substances synthesized in the central nervous system exert actions on the hormones and events associated with the menstrual cycle. The LH surge, and possibly ovulation, are facilitated by norepinephrine but inhibited by dopamine, and dopamine acts to reduce prolactin by active inhibition. The complexity of these interacting systems is further enhanced by the fact that the strength of these relationships is frequently dependent upon the basal levels of these various hormones.

3

The Impact
of Environmental Stressors
on the Menstrual Cycle

The physiological effects of stress are numerous, and considerable research has been devoted to this topic. This discussion will be limited to those physiological responses to stress that may interfere with or affect normal cyclic menstrual activity and those that may be of potential use in the understanding of certain gynecological disorders. Thus, this discussion will focus on the synthesis, release, and effects of neurotransmitters and hormones of the hypothalamus, the anterior pituitary, and the adrenal cortex with regard to responses to or covariates of stress. There is considerable clinical evidence regarding the effects of stress on menstrual cycle function and regulation: transient stressors, like the death of a friend, can induce anovulatory cycles and/or influence cycle duration; chronic stress can result during periods of amenorrhea; conflicts over pregnancy or the belief that one is pregnant can produce pseudocyesis; rape can trigger ovulation. The mechanisms by which psychological stress or beliefs are translated into physiological events has been the focus of much research.

Transient Stress

In a previous section, evidence was presented to suggest that levels of neurotransmitters in the central nervous system exerted an influence on menstrual activity, particularly those actions concerned with ovulation. The effects of stress on the synthesis and release of neurotransmitters, especially norepinephrine, have been the focus of much research. In general, psychological and/or physical stress tends to increase plasma levels of norepinephrine, epinephrine, dopamine, and serotonin (see, for example, Akiskal, 1979; Barnes et al., 1982; Dimsdale & Moss, 1980; Palmblad et al., 1977). In those studies that have measured more than one neurotransmitter during stress, it has been found that norepinephrine tends to be the most responsive of the three (Aslan et al., 1981; Mason et al., 1973; Woolf et al., 1983). Youngs and Reame (1983) have hypothesized that the enhanced catecholamine formation to stress results from a stress-induced increase in adrenal glucocorticoids that stimulate the production of tyrosine hydroxylase—the enzyme required for the rate-limiting step in the production of catecholamines. They also point out that stress in animals has been shown to decrease monoamine oxidase activity, which would serve to potentiate the action of brain catecholamines.

Since fluctuations in norepinephrine have typically been measured in the plasma, there has been some question as to whether or not these fluctuations represent levels of norepinephrine in the central nervous system. The metabolism of norepinephrine in the brain yields 3-methoxy-4-hydroxyphenylethylene glycol (MOPEG), which is excreted in the urine. Frankenhaeuser and colleagues (1978) measured changes in the excretion of this metabolite during periods of transient stress and consistently found significant correlations between plasma norepinephrine levels and urinary MOPEG. Furthermore, Sweeney and Maas (1979) reported that urinary MOPEG excretion covaried with state anxiety in a sample of acutely depressed female inpatients. Although MOPEG is also formed from the peripheral metabolism of norepinephrine, these data have been interpreted as indicating that the changes in plasma norepinephrine associated with stress do reflect levels of norepinephrine in the central nervous system.

Stress researchers have also extensively investigated responses to stress of the hypothalamic–pituitary–adrenal axis. The end product of the stress response of this system is cortisol—a glucocorticoid released from the adrenal cortex. The research is fairly consistent in indicating that stress results in increased levels of cortisol (see, for example, Hamanaka et al., 1970; Palmblad et al., 1977; Rahe, Rubin, & Arthur, 1974; Sowers et al., 1977). The mechanism by which cortisol is increased during periods of stress is initiated in the central nervous system. The hypothalamus releases corticotropin-releasing hormone (CRH) into the portal system, which supplies the anterior pituitary. In response to CRH, the pituitary secretes ACTH; and cortisol secretion by the adrenal cortex is controlled almost exclusively by ACTH.

Much of the early stress research was based on the assumption that the pituitary-adrenal cortical response to stress was a general one and did not vary with specific parameters associated with the stressor. Such assumptions were part of a widely accepted theory proposed by Selye (1950), which hypothesized a General Adaptation Syndrome consisting of a pattern of neuroendocrine changes to sustained arousal produced by a wide variety of stimuli. Selye defined stress as ". . . the nonspecific response of the body to any demand" (p. 55). Later researchers have taken issue with this theory and have suggested that there is considerable variability in physiological responses to stress, and such variability is a function of the individual's genetic make-up, learning history, and current physiological, social, and psychological states as well as specific characteristics of the stimulus situation (Engel, 1960; Steptoe, 1980). Within this context, changes in response to stress across the menstrual cycle have been studied. Although Abplanalp and colleagues (1977) found no evidence for significant variation in cortisol across phases of the menstrual cycle, Marinari, Leshner, and Doyle (1976) reported that women exposed to stressful situations during the premenstruum exhibited greater cortisol responses than did women tested at midcycle. These data suggest that the reactivity of the hypothalamic-pituitary-adrenal system may vary as a function of the menstrual cycle.

One recent refinement of stress theory has been to distinguish physiological consequences of the physical characteristics of the stimulus from those due to the psychological demands of the stimulus. Mason and coworkers (1976) studied the physiological responses of monkeys to fasting, exercise, and heat—all of which tend to produce a general arousal response similar to Selye's General Adaptation Syndrome. However, when presented in such a way as to eliminate the psychologically distressful components of the stimulus—by prevention of a hunger-induced uncomfortable stomach through provision of non-nutritive cellulose pellets and isolation of the monkeys to prevent them from watching others getting fed—the stress response was modified in the sense that there were no longer significant changes in corticosteroid levels in response to the stressors. These data are presented in Figure 3.1. Averill (1979) interpreted these findings to mean that this endocrine response, previously viewed as a nonspecific response to any stimulus, is

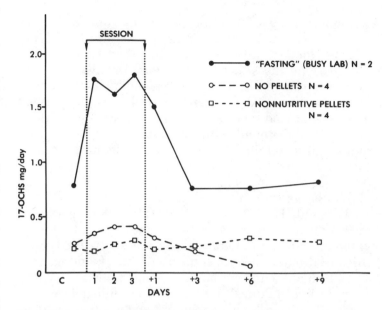

Figure 3.1. Urinary corticosteroid responses to three conditions of fasting in the monkey. (17-OHCS refers to 17-hydroxycorticosteroid, which is a by-product of cortisol metabolism; "busy lab" condition refers to monkeys who were deprived of food while housed with monkeys who were getting fed and who were not provided with non-nutritive pellets.)

Reprinted by permission from J. W. Mason, J. T. Maher, L. H. Hartley, E. H. Maugey, M. J. Perlow, and L. G. Jones, Selectivity of corticosteroid and catecholamine responses to various natural stimuli. In G. Serban (Ed.), *Psychopathology of Human Adaptation.* New York: Plenum, 1976.

instead a response specific to situations that have in common the ability to evoke psychological distress. Implicit in this theory is that learned or environmentally produced perceptual patterns or biases partially determine the specific stimuli an individual experiences as stressful and influence the degree, and perhaps the direction, of the physiological changes that occur in response to a stimulus (Burchfield, 1979).

The hypothalamic-pituitary-adrenal stress response appears to involve the release of substances in addition to those discussed above. Studies have found stress-induced increases in LH, growth hormone, and prolactin (Beardwood, Mundell, & Utian, 1975; Miyabo, Asato, & Mizushima, 1977; Noel et al., 1972; Sowers et al., 1977; Telner, Merali, & Singhal, 1982). In addition, Youngs and Reame

(1983) cite evidence to suggest that the endogenous opiates, endorphins, are released from the pituitary simultaneously with ACTH in response to stress. Not only are stress-induced endorphins useful in providing analgesia during situations that may involve pain, but related research suggests that endorphins may modulate the release of hormones in response to stress. Pontiroli and coworkers (1982) assessed the stress-induced increases in LH, prolactin, and cortisol with and without pretreatment with naloxone (an opiate antagonist); naloxone potentiated the LH rise, inhibited the prolactin elevation, and did not affect the cortisol response. Similarly, Quigley and Yen (1980) observed an increase in LH to nalozone, but only during late follicular and midluteal phases of the cycle.

Conversely, Reid, Hoff, and Yen (1981) noted a significant decrease in LH concentrations in men and women after administration of a synthetic endorphin. Others (Fritz & Speroff, 1983) have noted significant fluctuations in concentrations of endogenous opiates as a function of the menstrual cycle, with higher concentrations occurring during the luteal phase. Although integrating such diverse data is difficult without further systematic investigations, several tentative conclusions are possible: concentrations of several hormones of importance in the regulation of the menstrual cycle are altered during stress; endorphins seem to be involved in the release of these hormones; endorphin levels are influenced by stress and the phase of the menstrual cycle. Furthermore, it is tempting to speculate that, in addition to the hormonal influence on endogenous opiates, painful menstruation or the psychological stress associated with menstruation as a consequence of negative cultural values may result in increased levels of endorphins, which would, in turn, exert effects on LH and prolactin, and, ultimately, on the regulation of the menstrual cycle.

Chronic Stress

The studies discussed above were concerned with the effects of transient stressors, such as an examination, cold pressor, hunger, exercise, or shock. Other investigators have been interested in the physiological effects of chronic stress. Researchers have fairly consistently found that chronic stress results in depletion of central neurotransmitters, and, again, this effect is most pronounced with norepinephrine (Miller & Weiss, 1969; Seligman, 1975; Weiss et al., 1979). Attempting to integrate these opposing responses to transient and chronic stress in central neurotransmitter levels, Anisman (1978) has hypothesized the existence of two pools of norepinephrine—a newly synthesized pool and a storage pool. He suggests that mild transient stress promotes increased utilization of norepinephrine, which is compensated for by increased synthesis, and that MAO is partially inhibited, which reduces degradation of the newly formed catecholamines; in this way, the demands of the organism are met more than adequately, and there is a transient increase in norepinephrine. On the other hand, extremely intense and/or chronic stress increases the utilization of both the newly synthesized and the stored norepinephrine. Initially, this results in increased levels of brain amines via the process described above, but eventually, if the stress continues, synthesis cannot keep pace with utilization, and both newly synthesized and stored norepinephrine are depleted.

The relationship between norepinephrine and the hormonal and physical events surrounding ovulation are reviewed in the preceding chapter. To summarize, norepinephrine levels rise around the time of ovulation, and depletion of central catecholamines can result in a blunted or absent LH surge and anovulation. Thus, a reasonable, but tentative, hypothesis is that a possible cause of anovulatory menstrual cycles is chronic stress—the mediating mechanism being depletion of central norepinephrine stores. That severe, chronic stress is associated with anovulation and amenorrhea has been demonstrated in real-life situations—amenorrhea is common during war or incarceration in a concentration camp or prison; however, other factors of potential importance, such as malnutrition, generally play a part in such environments.

Empirical support for stress-induced anovulation is reported by Peyser and colleagues (1973). They admitted two healthy women, both with a history of regular ovulatory cycles, to the hospital, where they remained either for seven and ten days, respectively. Throughout their hospitalization, blood samples were obtained every 4 hours through an indwelling cannula. Although admitted to the hospital shortly before ovulation was expected, no LH surge occurred. Within 48 hours after being discharged from the hospital, both women exhibited a typical LH surge, which was at least a week delayed. That the delay in ovulation was a consequence of the stress associated with hospitalization and the blood sampling procedures was suggested by elevated cortisol levels during the hospital stay.

Predictability and Controllability

Since the most sophisticated theories of stress currently define stress in terms of its consequences on the organism, considerable research has been devoted to defining the parameters influencing those consequences. One such parameter has been the predictability of the stressor. Burchfield (1979), in an attempt to integrate relevant stress research, concluded that after repeated exposure to a stressor, the time course of adrenocortical secretion is altered so that the maximal response occurs prior to the stressor rather than during it—assuming that the stressor is temporally predictable. Depletion of central norepinephrine stores, resulting in a lack of transient norepinephrine elevations to discrete stressors, and maintenance of adrenocortical responding are not necessarily contradictory. Sachar (1980) has hypothesized that a noradrenergic system maintains a tonic inhibition of stress-induced ACTH secretion under normal conditions. However, when brain norepinephrine is depleted, this inhibition is lifted, and hypersecretion of ACTH and cortisol occurs. Thus, predictable chronic stress may be associated with central depletion of norepinephrine and enhanced cortisol responses.

Another stress parameter of considerable interest is controllability; that is, whether or not the individual has control or believes to have control over the stressor. The phenomenon of control has been of major interest to clinical psychologists for many years as the basis for the widely accepted theory of learned helplessness as a model of reactive depression; according to this model, reactive depression results when individuals experience a lack of control over important areas of their lives (Seligman, 1975). The interest in control has been extended to research concerned with the physiological consequences of stress. For example, Hanson, Larson, and Snowdon (1976) examined the effects of control over exposure to high-intensity noise on plasma cortisol levels in rhesus monkeys; plasma cortisol levels were significantly elevated in monkeys with no control and those experiencing a loss of control, while cortisol levels in animals with control did not differ from those in animals not exposed to noise.

Interested in the responses of cortisol and growth hormone to stress, Feldmann and Brown (1976) obtained plasma samples at regular intervals while rhesus monkeys were shocked and then given control over the shock by successfully learning to avoid the shock with a lever press. Both cortisol and growth hormone exhibited initial elevations, but activation of both hormones ceased when animals were well trained and able to avoid most of the shocks. In a related study, Frankenhaeuser (1976) measured adrenaline excretion in humans exposed to a series of tasks varying on a continuum of uncontrollable to complete mastery; adrenaline output decreased successively as the degree of control increased from helplessness to mastery. These data may be viewed in light of Averill's (1979) theory discussed above; perhaps, when a stressor is under an individual's control, the psychologically distressing aspects of the stimulus are eliminated, as is the associated physiological response.

Weiss and colleagues (1979) designed a series of studies in order to study the effect of control over stressors on behavior and brain catecholamines. Most of their experiments utilized an experimental design in which rats were tested in sets of three: one, called the avoidance-escape animal, was allowed to perform a response to terminate shocks or to avoid shocks; the second, called the yoked animal, received the same shocks as the avoidance-escape animal, but the animal did not have control over the shock; the third animal was a nonshock control. Of primary interest in these experiments was the comparison between the avoidance-escape animal and the yoked animal, since both received the same amount of shock and differed only on whether or not they had control over the shock. In an early experiment, they found that ". . . yoked animals showed depletions of brain norepinephrine as well as augmented uptake whereas avoidance-escape animals did not show these changes . . ." (p. 133).

Both Seligman and colleagues and Weiss and colleagues noted that animals exposed to chronic, inescapable shock exhibited behavioral deficits—that is, they became passive and were slow in learning future tasks. Seligman (1975) attributed this behavioral deficit to learning—the animals learned to be helpless and passive. In contrast, Weiss and coworkers (1979) concluded that animals exposed to uncontrollable stressors exhibit a depletion of brain norepinephrine and that it is these biochemical changes that interfere with the animals' ability to produce active behavior. To support their conclusions, they cite evidence to suggest that the depletion of norepinephrine by drugs resulted in a marked deficiency in avoidance-escape behavior. A second experiment by these authors, in which the administration of an MAO inhibitor prior to the inescapable shock prevented the behavioral deficits, provided further support for their hypothesis.

Similarly, the release of endogenous opiates has been related to stress and, specifically, to the dimension of controllability. Stress-induced analgesia is a recently discovered phenomenon that involves a decrease in pain sensitivity following exposure to a wide variety of stimuli that have in common the ability to elicit psychological distress. According to Maier and colleagues (1983), there are two forms of stress-induced analgesia (SIA)—one mediated by the release of endogenous opiates, the other mediated by nonopioid substances. In a series of four experiments by these authors, they found strong evidence to suggest that the dimensions of stress that are crucial in evoking opioid SIA are those of chronicity and uncontrollability; the animals exposed to chronic, uncontrollable shock exhibited opioid SIA—the opioid nature being assessed by the effectiveness of naloxone in blocking the effect—and the behavioral deficits typically seen with this procedure. Furthermore, Watkins and Mayer (1982) have concluded that opioid SIA can be classically conditioned, so that, like cortisol, endogenous opiates may be released prior to the stressor if the stressor is predictable.

One can infer from these data that it is not chronic stress per se that causes adrenal cortical activation, depletion of norepinephrine in the central nervous system, opioid SIA, and subsequent behavioral deficits, but chronic, uncontrollable stress. Furthermore, if the stressor is uncontrollable but predictable, the organism may exhibit an anticipatory stress response in the form of elevations in cortisol and endogenous opiates prior to the stressor. Although these inferences are tentative and the data amenable to alternative interpretations, the implications of these conclusions are potentially relevant to menstrual cycle symptomatology. Menstruation is a chronic and uncontrollable but predictable event and is stressful for some women. For those women who view menstruation as stressful, the literature reviewed here would suggest that, prior to menstruation, these women would exhibit lowered levels of central norepinephrine and elevations in endogenous opiates, covariates of depression, and heightened levels of cortisol, a covariate of tension and anxiety: and depression, tension, and anxiety are frequently reported as symptoms by women suffering from premenstrual syndrome.

Summary

The research on the physiological effects of stress indicates that the activity of the central nervous system and the hypothalamic-pituitary-adrenal system are highly sensitive to stress, as indicated by the changes in synthesis and release of the various neurochemicals produced by these systems. Furthermore, it is clear that there is considerable variability in response to stress and that the parameters influencing this variability, such as predictability and control, have only begun to be investigated. However, regardless of the subtleties involved in delineating the relevant parameters, the available research clearly indicates that stress influences levels of neurotransmitters in the central nervous system and that these, in turn, may well influence the rate of synthesis and release of hypothalamic releasing hormones, gonadotropins, and ovarian steroids. Thus, social–environmental stress may well play a role in the causation or exacerbation of such gynecological disorders as premenstrual tension, dysmenorrhea, amenorrhea, and menopausal hot flashes.

The influence of environmental stressors on the menstrual cycle leaves much of conventional methodology open to question. Traditional experimental design requires that one specify independent and dependent variables, assumed to be causes and effects, respectively. Much of the research on the menstrual cycle assumes the independent variables to be the phase of the menstrual cycle or hormonal levels and the dependent variables to be mood, behavior, or discomfort. The stress research indicates, however, that mood, behavior, or discomfort can be the causes and hormonal changes or changes in various characteristics of the menstrual cycle, such as the occurrence of ovulation or the length of the cycle, the effects; and these effects can, in turn, be causal of other processes or events. Thus, an appreciation and understanding of the potential for mutually interacting events are a prerequisite to the development of a more sophisticated and productive methodology for investigations concerned with the effects of stress on the menstrual cycle.

4

Covariates
of the Menstrual Cycle
in Normal Populations

"Edgar Berman, a physician and Democratic Party functionary . . . announced in 1970 that he would not like to see a woman in charge of this country at a time of national crisis because her 'raging hormonal imbalances' would threaten the life and safety of all" (Delaney, Lupton, & Toth, 1977, p. 48). Although rather extreme, Dr. Berman's views on women are consistent with the pervasive stereotypic concept of a woman's emotions and behaviors dictated by her hormonal state—she is irritable and depressed before menstruation, in pain and hysterical during menstruation, and "normal" only during the remainder of the month. There is no question that all normally menstruating women exhibit a relatively predictable pattern of hormonal fluctuations and some women experience psychological and/or physical stress associated with their menstrual cycle; but, as will become evident in the discussion below, the view that such distress is the inevitable and ubiquitous consequence of normal hormonal fluctuations is more a reflection of the myths and stereotypes surrounding women in our society and less a reflection of scientific fact.

In general, there is a lack of distinction, both theoretically and empirically, between menstrual disorders and a variety of normal physical, psychological, and behavioral changes that covary with the menstrual cycle. For example, findings indicative of covariation between depression and progesterone in a group of women diagnosed as suffering from premenstrual syndrome do not imply that all women's moods covary with progesterone levels; conversely, data suggesting that, in a random sample of normal women, there is not a significant increase in pain during menstruation should not be viewed as evidence that dysmenorrhea is not a distressing and debilitating problem for some women. In this chapter, research concerned with changes in physical, psychological, and behavioral variables during the menstrual cycle in random samples of normal women will be reviewed and critically analyzed. Prior to this discussion, however, several issues relevant to the methodology of menstrual cycle research will be addressed.

Methodological Issues in Menstrual Cycle Research

The Measurement of Menstrual Cycle Covariates

During the past several decades, one area of interest to researchers has been the assessment of emotional states, physical discomfort, and psychological variables as fluctuating with the menstrual cycle. With the increasing emphasis on a "scientific" approach, there has been a shift away from interview techniques, which are viewed as potentially subjective and biased, to standardized tests that are viewed as being free of bias, useful for "objective" assessment, and, if well designed, reliable and valid. Two instruments have been developed in attempts to provide a reliable and valid assessment of variables that are thought to covary with the menstrual cycle: The Menstrual Symptom Questionnaire and the Menstrual Distress Questionnaire.

The Menstrual Symptom Questionnaire (MSQ) was developed by Chesney and Tasto (1975a) and was theoretically derived from Dalton's (1964) distinction between spasmodic symptoms—spasms of pain that begin on the first day of menstruation—and congestive symptoms—dull, aching pain accompanied by lethargy and depression prior to menstruation. These categories are conceptually and empirically similar to the more commonly used terms of dysmenorrhea and premenstrual syndrome, respectively. According to Dalton, the former is due to an excess of progesterone, the latter to insufficient progesterone; thus, according to this theory, it is unlikely that one individual would experience both.

The purposes of the MSQ were to distinguish between these two types of symptoms and to provide a score indicative of the severity of the symptoms. Chesney and Tasto (1975a) obtained 51 items from the literature; each was rated on a five-point scale, which reflected the degree to which the symptom was present. Their first sample consisted of 56 women who stated that they experienced menstrual discomfort. A factor analysis resulted in two factors on which 25 of the items loaded. These two factors conformed somewhat to the definitions of spasmodic and congestive dysmenorrhea. Data from a second sample of 48 subjects essentially replicated those of the first group.

Since these authors assumed that both types of symptoms did not occur in the same woman, they developed a scoring procedure that reversed the scoring for spasmodic items, resulting in high scores being indicative of a spasmodic disorder and low scores of a congestive disorder. In other words, women received high scores if they endorsed spasmodic items but not congestive items and low scores if they endorsed congestive items but not spasmodic items. Since the authors assumed that any particular woman does not suffer from both disorders, this scoring procedure did not allow for a distinction between women who experienced neither set of symptoms and women who experienced both. Chesney and Tasto (1975a) reported a test–retest reliability coefficient of .87, and Cox (1977) reported similar results. In addition, Chesney and Tasto (1975b) found differential treatment effectiveness for the two types of symptoms using behavior modification techniques. Cox (1977) and Cox and Meyer (1978), however, found behavioral therapy to be equally effective for spasmodic and congestive disorders.

Criticism of the MSQ has come from several sources. Data from Cox (1977) raised doubts as to the discriminative validity of the instrument. He found that the mean score of a group of women who complained of menstrual distres was almost identical to that of a group who claimed to experience no distress. Probably the most serious criticism of the MSQ came from Webster and colleagues (1979). Claiming that Chesney and Tasto's sample was too small for their statistical techniques, they performed a hypothesis-testing factor analysis on data from 275 subjects. Ten of the 12 spasmodic items correlated significantly with the spasmodic factor, and four of the 12 congestive items correlated with the congestive factor. Thus, 10 of the 24 items did not load as predicted, and the original factors were not supported. Furthermore, if Dalton (1964) was correct and the two disorders are mutually exclusive, then spasmodic and congestive scores should be inversely related. The correlation coefficient between the two scores was .56, indicating not only that it is possible for the two disorders to occur together but that it is likely that they do. The results of these studies not only raise doubts as to the validity of the MSQ but question the soundness of the theoretical base as well.

Far more popular has been the Menstrual Distress Questionnaire (MDQ) developed by Moos (1968, 1977), which was designed to evaluate menstruation-related symptoms during premenstrual, menstrual, and intermenstrual phases of the cycle. The questionnaire consists of 47 symptoms, which were initially obtained from interviews with women and from previous research in the area of menstrual cycle symptomatology. In addition, symptoms not typically associated with the menstrual cycle, such as buzzing or ringing in the ears and feelings of suffocation, were included in order to obtain a measure of general complaining. Of the 47 symptoms, only 4 are positive—affection, excitement, feelings of well-being, and bursts of energy or activity. A six-point scale, which rates severity from "no experience of symptoms" to "acute or partially disabling," accompanies each symptom.

In the initial sample of 839 wives of graduate students, each subject completed four questionnaires rating symptoms for the menstrual (during flow), premenstrual (the week prior to flow), and intermenstrual (the rest of the cycle) phases of her most recent menstrual cycle and of her worst menstrual cycle. Data from each phase were factor analyzed separately and resulted in eight symptom groups. All items, except change in eating habits, loaded consistently on a factor. Moos labeled the scales as follows: pain, water retention, concentration, negative affect, behavior change, arousal, autonomic reaction, and control. All the positive items loaded on the arousal scale. Pain, concentration, behavior change, and autonomic reactions were higher during the menstrual than the premenstrual phase, while the reverse was true for water retention and negative affect; all these scales were lowest during the intermenstrual phase. The arousal and control scales did not show cyclic variation. Unfortunately, Moos did not report statistics for these cyclic effects, so it is difficult to determine the reliability of the phase differences for these scales.

Later research employing the MDQ to measure differences in menstrual symptomatology among different phases of the cycle has yielded mixed results. For example, Golub (1976a) found negative affect, concentration, and behavior change to be significantly higher premenstrually than intermenstrually. Gruba and Rohrbaugh (1975) found significant differences between all pairs of menstrual, premenstrual, and intermenstrual comparisons for all scales except arousal, and Parlee (1980) noted that her subjects reported higher levels of negative affect during premenstrual and menstrual phases than during the rest of the cycle.

Others have used Form T of the MDQ, the original form modified to assess symptoms on a daily basis ("indicate how you feel today"). Using this form, Wilcoxon, Schrader, and Sherif (1976) showed that four of the eight scales differed significantly among phases, while in a more recent study (Doty et al., 1981) only two—pain and water retention—exhibited significant phase effects. Silbergeld, Brast, and Noble (1971) analyzed each item and each scale for phase effects and found one scale and three items to vary significantly—approximately what one would expect by chance.

Moos (1977) provided intercorrelations for the eight scales for each phase; all were positive, with a range of .18 to .63, indicating that women who scored high on one scale also scored high on other scales, including the control scale. He also intercorrelated the three cycle phases for each scale; again, all the correlation coefficients were positive, ranging from .17 to .77, an indication that women tended to endorse the same symptoms in all three phases. Parlee (1974) pointed out that these interscale and interphase correlations suggest that a response bias may be operating—that is, the questionnaire may be measuring a tendency to respond high or low, regardless of the content of the item. This suggestion receives further support when one considers that Moos and colleagues (1969) reported a small but positive correlation between arousal, which consists of positive items, and all other scales, which consist of negative items.

An important requirement for any assessment procedure is reliability. Markum (1976) assessed split-half reliability for each scale of the MDQ and for each phase; all were significant, with all but one correlation coefficient being above .80. She also analyzed both forms of the MDQ, retrospective and daily, for intercycle stability for all scales and the three phases. All correlations were high (.41 to .96), except for the total score and the arousal scale on the daily form for the menstrual phase, which were .26 and .20, respectively. Moos and coworkers (1969) studied 15 women for two cycles on 24 of the items and found generally high correlations (.39 to .95). These studies suggest that the MDQ is a fairly reliable instrument.

Several researchers have questioned the validity of the original form of the MDQ, Form A, on the basis that it is a retrospective questionnaire and relies on memory. A possible test of this criticism would be to administer both Form A and Form T to the same women and compare the responses. Moos and colleagues (1969) selected two groups of women—one high on premenstrual tension, the other low on premenstrual tension—on the basis of their responses to Form A. They then administered Form T to these women for two consecutive cycles. Nine of the 15 women showed consistency between Form A and Form T. In a later study, Rouse (1978) reported significant differences between the two forms on pain, water retention, and negative affect scales, with the retrospective form eliciting greater reporting of distress than the daily form. Finally, Brockway (1975) administered Form A and, on the basis of these data, formed three groups, which were low, moderate, and high on premenstrual symptoms. The subjects then completed Form T daily for two cycles. Brockway analyzed the water retention, pain, and negative affect scales and found significant differences between Forms A and T for all groups and all scales, except for the low-symptom group on water retention.

Several studies have compared responses on the retrospective form of the MDQ to a daily assessment of symptoms utilizing a different instrument. Schilling (1981) administered the retrospective form of the MDQ and a daily mood checklist. Significant correlations were not found between MDQ negative affect and a daily assessment of sadness, between MDQ pain and daily assessment of sickness, and between MDQ concentration and a daily assessment of concentration; there was, however, a significant correlation between MDQ arousal and a daily assessment of surgency. Interestingly, Parlee (1980) found significantly higher levels of negative affect during premenstrual and menstrual phases of the cycle as assessed by the retrospective form of the MDQ, but, on a different instrument administered daily, the same women reported premenstrual elation. In general, these studies indicate that the reported degree of menstruation-related distress partially depends upon whether symptoms are assessed on a retrospective or daily basis and that a greater amount of distress is reported on retrospective questionnaires than on those that assess symptoms on a daily basis.

Differences in retrospective and daily reporting of symptoms may result from the influence of cultural stereotypes on a woman's reporting of menstrual symptoms; that is, it is generally believed that women are moody or irritable prior to menses and suffer from incapacitating pain during menses. Thus, women who experience minimal symptoms or none may exaggerate their responses when reporting retrospectively (Brooks-Gunn & Ruble, 1979; Parlee, 1974; Ruble, 1977). Parlee (1974) administered the MDQ to 25 women and 34 men, with instructions to complete one questionnaire for each of the three phases according to their experience with, or knowledge of, these symptoms. The data from both groups showed significant phase effects for most scales. In all but one of the 24 instances (eight scales, three phases), men gave greater severity ratings than did the women; these differences were statistically significant in 11 cases. Parlee concluded that the stereotypic beliefs act to exaggerate the actual, experienced symptomatology when reported on retrospective questionnaires.

Another method of assessing the effect of stereotypic beliefs on the reporting of symptomatology related to the menstrual cycle is to compare responses from persons who are aware that the intent of the questionnaire is to evaluate menstrual symptoms and responses from those who believe that the purpose of the questionnaire is to evaluate general health. Rogers and Harding (1981) administered the MDQ to 136 women and 104 men; half of the women and all of the men received a version with the word "menstrual" removed from the title. All were asked to report on symptoms for the previous seven days (menstrual), 7 to 17 days prior (premenstrual), and 14 to 35 days prior (midcycle). No significant differences were found in total distress among the three groups during menstrual and premenstrual phases; however, during the midcycle phase, women receiving the informed version reported significantly less distress than the other two groups. Since menstrual symptoms must, by definition, exhibit changes across phases of the cycle, only the scores of the informed group were indicative of menstrual symptoms; the uninformed women and the men reported symptoms, but not symptoms that varied with the menstrual cycle. Although the informed women were the only group to have shown cyclic changes, they also reported significantly less total distress across all phases than did the other two groups.

In a similar study, Chernovetz, Jones, and Hansson (1979) gave the MDQ to 60 women and 58 men; half of each sex were uninformed as to the menstrual nature of the questionnaire (the informed men were told that the authors were interested in determining whether menstrual-like symptoms occurred in men). Subjects were also asked to provide a general rating of their over-all health. Total MDQ scores were, as in the study above, higher for subjects who were ignorant of the menstrual context. Total MDQ scores and health ratings were unrelated for the informed subjects but were significantly correlated among subjects who were uninformed.

From these two studies one can infer that if persons believe that menstruation-related symptoms are being assessed, they will only attend to symptoms that coincide in content and timing with the stereotyped view of menstrual symptoms and ignore symptoms not typically believed to be related to menstruation and time periods (midcycle) during which menstrual symptoms are believed not to occur. For example, an informed subject confronted with a question referring to backache may consider only whether she had a backache before or during her period, while an uninformed subject may consider whether she had a backache at any time during the month. Such an interpretation is a logical, but empirically unverified, explanation for the finding that uninformed women reported greater total distress but fewer phase-related symptoms than did informed women. Also, as pointed out by Ruble and Brooks-Gunn (1979), the cultural stereotype, manifested as an individual's perceptual bias, may result in a particular behavior or feeling being labelled differently, depending upon its temporal relationship to the cycle; for example, a particular sensation may be labelled as indigestion if it occurs during the midcycle but as cramps if it occurs during menstruation.

The existence of such cultural stereotypes regarding the debilitating effects of menstruation has been demonstrated in a study by Golub (1981). She questioned both men and women concerning their beliefs regarding menstruation; 75% of the men, but only 32% of the women stated that women's thinking is affected by menstruation; over half of both groups believed that women do not function as well when menstruating and that a woman's personality changes during menstruation. Furthermore, evidence that such cultural stereotypes influence the reporting of menstrual symptoms comes from a study, unique for its creative design, by Ruble (1977). Women subjects were told that it is now scientifically possible to predict the date of their next period. Subjects were given fake brain wave tests; then a third of the subjects were told that their period was not expected for seven to ten days, a third that their period was due in one or two days, and a third was given no information. (All subjects were actually tested about one week prior to their period.) They were then asked to fill out the MDQ on the basis of symptoms they had experienced in the last day or two. Ruble analyzed three of the eight scales. The water retention, pain, and negative affect scales were higher for those women who believed they were premenstrual than for those who believed they were intermenstrual; differences in the first two scales reached statistical significance. Ruble suggests that learned associations or beliefs may result in women exaggerating their actual experience.

Matthews and Carra (1982) hypothesized that certain personality characteristics would interact with cultural stereotypes in determining the reporting of menstrual symptoms. They postulated that women designated as Type A, defined as individuals who are highly motivated to achieve and perform well, would be motivated to ignore symptoms experienced during the menstrual flow because of the belief in the debilitating effects of menstrual symptoms on their performance. It was also predicted that these same women would not be motivated to ignore symptoms reported retrospectively, since these would not interfere with their current performance, nor those reported on a postmenstrual day, since, at this time, cultural stereotypes dictate that women experience a heightened functioning. Forty women completed a questionnaire measuring Type A behavior and an MDQ describing symptoms during a typical menstruation; the subjects were then asked to wait until the second day of their forthcoming menses and complete a daily form of the MDQ and another MDQ one week later. A series of partial correlations between menstrual symptoms and Type A behavior, adjusting for the retrospective and postmenstrual MDQ scores, revealed that ". . . relative to symptom intensity reported for either of the two comparison intervals, the more extreme the Type A behavior of women, the lower the intensity of symptoms reported during menstruation" (p. 149).

In summary, neither of the standardized instruments described above completely meets the need of researchers for a reliable and valid instrument for the assessment of menstruation-related symptoms. In addition to the problems discussed above, a further criticism of both instruments is their concentration on negative symptoms. Israel (1953) pointed out that women frequently report increased energy and feelings of well-being prior to menstruation, and Parlee (1980) noted that her subjects reported an increase in elation during the premenstruum. In research that aims to investigate physical, psychological, and behavioral changes that covary with the menstrual cycle, the emphasis on negative events and psychological processes seems unjustified and may act to perpetuate stereotypic beliefs concerning women.

Of the two, the MDQ seems preferable in that it has, at least, face validity. However, the MDQ, particularly Form A, may not be appropriate for use in research where the goal is to assess menstrual cycle symptoms in samples of normal women. It does not consistently differentiate between cycle phases, although this probably reflects a lack of cyclic variability in the normal population. Furthermore, the MDQ appears to be unacceptably sensitive to response biases, demand characteristics, and belief systems, unless the woman being assessed is unaware of the menstrual nature of the questionnaire.

The Determination
of Menstrual Cycle Phases

Menstrual cycle research has focused on the covariation of the menstrual cycle, with numerous aspects of physiological, endocrinological, psychological, behavioral, and physical changes related both to healthy and to disordered reproductive activity. Central to the theoretical interpretation of this research is the validity of the assumed fluctuations in circulating levels of estrogen and progesterone during the menstrual cycle. Since hormonal assays are time-consuming and expensive, some researchers have employed indirect and inexact procedures to determine hormonal levels.

As the levels of these hormones are time-locked to ovulation, some researchers have indirectly determined the time of ovulation and then assumed that, prior to this time, estrogen levels are high and progesterone levels minimal and that, subsequent to this time, levels of both estrogen and progesterone are high. In ovulatory cycles, these assumptions are appropriate; however, methods for determining the time of ovulation vary in their accuracy. The most common method utilizes the date of the last menses, the normal length of the cycle, and the predicted date of the next menses; ovulation is assumed to occur approximately 14 days prior to the onset of menses. This procedure is based on the widespread belief that the length of the menstrual cycle varies directly with the preovulatory phase, while the postovulatory phase is an invariant 14 days. Marshall (1963) ascertained the time of ovulation by basal temperature fluctuations and found that only 67% of 155 women exhibited a postovulatory phase of between 11 and 14 days. In a later study, Abplanalp and colleagues (1977) measured estrogen and progesterone concentrations and concluded that pinpointing ovulation on the basis of the dates of past and expected periods was successful in 50% of the cases. Thus, the self-report method of determining the time of ovulation has questionable validity.

A more objective method is that of recording basal temperature on a daily basis. It is believed that basal temperature increases slightly, but noticeably, at the time of ovulation and remains elevated until menses. Although this method is widely used not only by researchers but by women who wish to avoid or facilitate pregnancy, Sommer (1973) noted that only 25% of all women exhibit a clear temperature change at ovulation. Furthermore, Southam and Gonzaga (1965) compared dates of ovulation determined by endometrial and ovarian histology and basal temperature and reported as much as a four-day discrepancy between the two procedures.

Another common research procedure has been to divide the menstrual cycle into several phases and compare these phases on some criterion measure of interest, such as psychological depression or reaction time. Several problems are inherent in this procedure. Since the length of the menstrual cycle varies considerably among different women and within the same woman, a particular phase will vary in the length of time it represents. A common solution to this problem has been to designate the phases of primary interest as fixed and the phase of least interest as variable. For example, Dalton (1968) labeled the four days preceding menses as the premenstrual phase, the four days following onset as the menstrual phase, and the remainder of the phase as the intermenstrual phase. Unfortunately, no standard procedure exists for phase differentiation and definition; the consequence has been a tremendous amount of methodological variability in research related to the menstrual cycle. According to Sommer (1973), who presented an extensive tabulation of the idiosyncratic research procedures, the number of differentiated phases varied between one and seven. In addition, the definition of the same phase has varied from study to study; for example, the premenstrual phase has been designated as two days (Pierson & Lockhart, 1963), four days (Dalton, 1968), five days (Dalton, 1960b), and seven days (Sommer, 1972) prior to menstruation. Clearly, such procedural variability makes comparisons among studies difficult.

Summary

The contradictions and inconsistencies that characterize much of the research concerned with menstrual disorders and the menstrual cycle are at least partially due to the use of less-than-adequate methods for pinpointing the time of ovulation, to the lack of standardized procedures for defining cycle phases, to the lack of reliable and valid procedures for assessing menstruation-related symptoms, and to the influence of cultural stereotypes on the formulation of research hypotheses and methodologies. The reader is requested to keep these limitations in mind when considering the research presented in the following chapters.

Physical Covariates
of the Menstrual Cycle

The physical variables most commonly evaluated with respect to the menstrual cycle are pain, water retention, and weight gain. With regard to pain, researchers typically have predicted that abdominal pain will be greatest during menses and that pain associated with swelling of the breasts and extremities will peak premenstrually. In developing the Menstrual Distress Questionnaire (MDQ), Moos (1968) named one of his scales "pain," including muscle stiffness, headache, cramps, backache, fatigue, and general aches and pains. In the original sample of 839 women, this scale was higher menstrually than premenstrually and higher premenstrually than intermenstrually, although Moos did not report whether these differences were statistically significant.

In other studies, which have assessed differences in pain as a function of the phase of the menstrual cycle, the results appear to be dependent upon whether pain is assessed daily or in a retrospective fashion. In three studies (Abplanalp, Donnelly, & Rose, 1979; Gruba & Rohrbaugh, 1975; Rogers & Harding, 1981), retrospective forms of the MDQ were administered to normally menstruating women; they were told to complete three questionnaires by describing their previous menstrual, premenstrual, and intermenstrual phases. The results were similar for all three studies and indicated significant phase effects for the pain scale, with the menstrual phase being higher than the other phases.

On the other hand, when pain has been assessed on a daily basis throughout the menstrual cycle, either using the MDQ (Lahmeyer, Miller, & DeLeon-Jones, 1982; Markum, 1976; Swandby, 1981) or with a daily rating of pain (Janowsky, Berens, & Davis, 1973; Zimmerman & Parlee, 1973), pain has not been found to vary significantly across phases of the menstrual cycle. A study by Wilcoxon, Schrader, and Sherif (1976) is the only study utilizing a daily assessment of pain to have found significantly greater pain during menstruation than during the rest of the cycle. In a final note related to pain as covarying with the menstrual cycle, both Swandby (1981) and Rogers and Hardig (1981) included a sample of men in their studies of the menstrual cycle. Both used the MDQ, the daily and retrospective forms, respectively, and in neither study were there significant gender differences on the pain scale.

Thus, there is minimal evidence to suggest that, in a random sample of normally menstruating women, pain is experienced to a significantly greater extent during menstruation than during other phases of the cycle. Furthermore, the results of these studies are consistent with research discussed in a previous section, in which it was concluded that retrospective reports of symptoms tend to exaggerate symptomatology and probably reflect the influence of cultural stereotypes and attitudes and that daily reports are probably a more valid assessment of actual symptoms.

Other physical symptoms include swelling and weight gain, which tend to contribute to the discomfort experienced by women who complain of premenstrual syndrome. Studies of variables assumed to be associated with these symptoms have yielded contradictory, usually negative findings when subjects were drawn from a normal population. One of the scales on the MDQ is water retention, which consists of weight gain, skin disorders, painful breasts, and swelling. Moos (1968) found these items to be highest during the premenstruum. Gruba and Rohrbaugh (1975), Wilcoxon, Shrader, and Sherif (1976), Rogers and Harding (1981), Abplanalp, Donnelly, and Rose (1979), Lahmeyer, Miller, and DeLeon-Jones (1982), and Swandby (1981) found significant phase effects for water retention, which peaked during the premenstruum, and which was measured with either the retrospective or the daily form of the MDQ.

Studies utilizing objective measures of water retention, however, have generally failed to find similar results. Janowsky, Berens, and Davis (1973) found weight and potassium–sodium ratio to vary with the phase of the menstrual cycle, with both increasing premenstrually, while Gray and colleagues (1968) found no phase effects for potassium–sodium ratio. Andersch and coworkers (1978) did not find weight to vary with the menstrual cycle but did note a slight variation in total body water. Abramson and Torghele (1961) reported that similar peaks in weight occurred on days 3–6, 13–15, and 24–26; they viewed these weight fluctuations as significant but did not present statistics. An average weight fluctuation of 0.7 pounds was reported for 69 subjects by Golub, Menduke, and Conly (1965), and the subjects differed as to where in the cycle they weighed the most. Finally, Wong and colleagues (1972) measured the capillary filtration coefficent as an index of the flow of fluid from the intravascular to the extravascular compartment and reported no significant variation attributable to the menstrual cycle in normal women.

In summary, research assessing menstrual cycle variability in physical variables associated with common menstrual complaints of pain and swelling or weight gain has yielded inconsistent results. The fact that retrospective or self-report measures typically have yielded stronger results than daily or objective measures suggests either that women are reporting their expectations rather than their experiences or that the relevant variables are not being assessed. Consistent use and reporting of statistical analyses would certainly aid interpretation; however, the research to date suggests that these physical variables show minimal fluctuations with the menstrual cycle in samples of normal women.

Psychological Covariates
of the Menstrual Cycle

That a woman's psychological state fluctuates with her menstrual cycle is a commonly held belief, although the soundness of the scientific evidence for these fluctuations has been questioned (Parlee, 1973). Clinical reports have suggested that negative psychological states are a major complaint of women with menstrual disorders, particularly those suffering from premenstrual syndrome (Israel, 1967). According to Moos's (1968) factor analysis of the MDQ, negative affect was one of eight coherent factors. This scale consists of crying, loneliness, anxiety, restlessness, irritability, mood swings, depression, and tension. In Moos's original sample, negative affect was higher during the premenstruum and menses than during the intermenstruum. However, statistical tests of these differences were not reported, and the retrospective form of the MDQ was used.

Twenty studies investigating the relationship between the menstrual cycle and psychological symptoms, not assessed retrospectively, are summarized in Table 4.1. It should be pointed out that many of these studies included other measures and/or other groups, but only psychological measures in normal unmedicated women are reported in the table. Most of the instruments are self-explanatory, with the exception of the G–GFAT, which refers to the Gottschalk–Gleser Free Association Test. In this test, subjects are

Table 4.1

Studies Relating Psychological Variables to the Menstrual Cycle

Study	Number of Subjects	Measures	Results
Abplanalp, Livingston, Rose, & Sandwisch (1977)	21	State-Trait Anxiety Inventory. Half of subjects tested during menses, half during midcycle.	No significant differences.
Abplanalp, Rose, Donnelly, & Livingston-Vaughan (1979)	14	Profile of Mood States and Social-Sexual Activities. Log daily for 2 cycles.	No relationship between mood states or enjoyment of activities and phase of the menstrual cycle.
Beaumont, Richards, & Gelder (1975)	25	Symptom check list daily for 1 cycle. Scored for negative mood.	Significant cyclic variation in mood. Higher negative mood premenstrually and menstrually than intermenstrually.
Dan (1980)	24	G-GFAT* scored for anxiety and hostility and rated activation, hostility, depression, anger and frustration. Twice a week for 2 months.	No significant phase effects.

Study	N	Method	Results
Golub (1976b)	50	Depression Adjective Check List, MDQ, State-Trait Anxiety Inventory. Tested 4 days prior to menses and 2 weeks after menses.	Significant cycle effects for depression and state anxiety with premenstruum higher than midcycle.
Gottschalk, Kaplan, Gleser, & Wingest (1962)	5	G-GFAT* scored for anxiety and 3 measures of hostility. Tested 5–7 times/week for 1–3 cycles.	Analyzed data for individual subjects. Of the 20 analyses, 5 were significant. Of these 5, 3 peaked during premenstruum.
Halbreich & Kas (1977)	22	Taylor Manifest Anxiety Scale. 4 times in 1 cycle.	No significant phase effects.
Ivey & Bardwick (1968)	26	G-GFAT* scored for anxiety. Tested at ovulation and premenstruum for cycles.	Premenstrual anxiety significantly higher than ovulatory.
Lahmeyer, Miller, & Deleon-Jones (1982)	11	MDQ, State-Trait Anxiety Inventory daily for 1 cycle.	No significant phase effects.
Little & Zahn (1974)	12	Nowlis Mood Adjective Check List 6 days/week for 1 cycle.	No significant phase effects for negative mood scale scores.
Marinari, Leshner, & Doyle (1976)	60	Rated depressed, confused, embarrassed, confident, cheerful, anxious, excitable, apathetic after stressor either premenstrually or midcycle.	No significant differences.

(continued)

Table 4.1 *(continued)*

Study	Number of Subjects	Measures	Results
Paige (1971)	38	G-GFAT* scored for hostility and anxiety. Combined for total negative affect. Tested on days 4, 10, 16, and 26 of 1 cycle.	Significant decrease in all three measures between days 4 to 16. Significant increase in total negative affect and hostility between days 16 and 26.
Parlee (1980)	7	Thayer Activation–Deactivation Adjective Check List and Profile of Mood States daily for 90 days.	Depression–dejection, fatigue, de-activation-sleep, and confusion significantly lower during premenstrual than ovulatory phase. Confusion and anger-hostility significantly lower during menstrual than ovulatory phase.
Patkai, Johannson, & Post (1974)	6	Verbal attitudes towards words *I, man, woman,* and *sex.* Scored for brisk, tense, concentrated, apprehensive, irritable, efficient, gloomy, restless. Tested 5 days/week for 1–2 cycles.	Apprehensive and restless, showed significant cycle effects. Peak restlessness was premenstrual, peak apprehension was postmenstrual.

Rogers & Harding (1981)	14	MDQ-Form T. Once during mid-cycle phase and once during premenstrual phase.	Negative affect significantly higher premenstrually than during mid-cycle.
Schilling (1981)	27	Mood Adjective Check List daily for 35 days.	No significant phase effects.
Silbergeld, Brast, & Noble (1971)	8	MDQ (Form T), Mood Adjective Check List, half-hour unstructured interview. 9 times during 1 cycle.	Analyzed 138 variables in separate analyses. 8 showed significant phase effects (expect 7 by chance).
Swandby (1981)	8	Multiple Affect Adjective Check List and MDQ-Form T daily for 35 days.	Difficulty in concentration significantly higher during ovulatory phase than during the rest of the cycle.
Wilcoxon, Schrader, & Sherif (1976)	11	Pleasant Activities Schedule, MDQ (Form T), Mood Adjective Check List, Personal Stress Inventory. Daily for 1 cycle.	Assessed negative affect, impaired concentration, and number of stressful events. All 3 variables showed significant cycle effects peaking during premenstruum.
Zimmerman & Parlee (1973)	14	Anxiety, fear, depression, irritability. Rated daily for 1 cycle.	No significant phase effects.

*Gottschalk-Gleser Free Association Test.

requested to speak for five minutes about any memorable experience in their lives. The verbal content of the speech is then analyzed for death anxiety, mutilation anxiety, separation anxiety, guilt anxiety, shame anxiety, diffuse anxiety, total anxiety, hostility outwards-overt, hostility outwards-covert, hostility inwards, ambivalent hostility, and total hostility.

Of the 20 studies listed, one involved numerous analyses, and the number of significant results approximated what one would expect by chance; four reported equivocal results in the sense that significance was achieved, but the differences were not consistently in the hypothesized direction; six reported statistically significant phase effects in the predicted direction; and nine failed to find phase effects. Several of these studies require additional comment. Golub (1976b), who found elevated depression and anxiety scores during the premenstruum, compared these scores to the scores of subjects in other research studies. Although one can only speculate when comparing data from independent studies, she noted that the premenstrual depression scores were lower than those reported by psychiatric patients, similar to those of pregnant women in the first trimester, and higher than those of normal women college students. The premenstrual state anxiety scores were lower than those of students undergoing the mild stress of freshman orientation or a class examination. Golub concluded that, although the phase effects were statistically significant, they were probably not clinically significant.

In the study by Wilcoxon, Schrader, and Sherif (1976), subjects recorded stressful events in their daily lives, as well as symptoms and moods. An analysis of the stress data revealed that the negative affect variables and impaired concentration were associated to a significantly greater extent with stressful events than with the phase of the menstrual cycle. This result diminishes the importance of menstrual cycle phase as a determinant of mood but leaves one trying to explain the increase in stressful events occurring during the premenstruum. One possible explanation is that during the premenstruum a woman may evaluate events as more stressful or react more to stressful events than during other times. Little and Zahn (1974) presented data that suggest cyclic variation in autonomic responsivity, but the peak of responsivity occurred around ovulation rather than premenstrually.

A frequent criticism of menstrual cycle research is that the size and clinical significance of the effects could be more realistically appraised if a control group of men were included. This was done in three of the studies included in the table. Parlee (1980) compared her results to those of an identical study of eight men and found women to exhibit fluctuations on significantly fewer scales than did the men. A group of 20 men were included in the study by Rogers and Harding (1981). There was not a significant sex difference in total distress scores from the MDQ; however, women exhibited significantly more variability in pain and men exhibited significantly more variability in behavior than did persons of the opposite gender. Finally, Swandby (1981) found mean mood scale scores to be nearly equivalent for men and women, and neither group demonstrated significant mood fluctuations as a function of the menstrual cycle for the women or of a 28-day cycle for the men.

Suicide is usually assumed to be associated with a negative psychological state, so the research on suicide and the menstrual cycle is included in this section. Three studies (Dalton, 1959b; Mandell & Mandell, 1967; Wetzel, McClure, & Reich, 1971) have reported a greater number of suicide attempts during menstruation than during other times in the cycle. A methodological flaw in these studies is that they relied on retrospective reporting to determine the phase of the cycle, and women unable to remember when their last period began were usually eliminated from the samples. This procedure would clearly bias the results in the sense that women who were menstruating would be more likely to remember when their period began than women who were not menstruating, and, thus, menstruating women would be more likely to be included in the studies. On the other hand, Tonks, Rack, and Rose (1968) found the highest rate of suicide attempts to be in the premenstruum; however, again they relied on retrospective reporting of phase. Similar studies have been reported by Birtchnell and Floyd (1974) and Holding and Minkoff (1973), who did not find significant phase effects for suicide attempts.

The only study of suicide and the menstrual cycle not relying on retrospective reporting of cycle phase was reported by MacKinnon, MacKinnon, and Thomson (1959), who determined the phase of the menstrual cycle by postmortem examination of the uterus. They determined the frequency of deaths occurring during various phases of the menstrual cycle in 102 women who died from suicide, disease, or accident. Sixty deaths occurred during the midluteal phase (6–13 days prior to menstruation). Although they did not report separate statistics for the different causes of death, their graphs suggested that the phase differences were marked for death resulting from suicide and disease but not for those due to accidents. Thus, the research on suicide and the menstrual cycle has not consistently placed high suicide rates in any one particular phase.

The study least subject to criticism on methodological grounds reported the highest rate to be during the midluteal phase, and these results applied to death by disease as well as to death by suicide.

Koeske (1980) has critically analyzed the research concerned with the study of psychological changes associated with the menstrual cycle. Her criticisms include the following: (1) the emphasis is on negative variables (hostility, anxiety, depression) to the exclusion of positive ones, and there is an underlying assumption, implicit in the interpretation of research results, that variables covarying with the menstrual cycle are causally related to biochemical imbalances; (2) researchers have neglected the potentially potent effects of environmental variables and stress both on the biochemical processes that may influence cycle length and on the psychological variables; (3) researchers have failed to separate beliefs and stereotypes about cycle-related emotionality from the causes of that emotionality; (4) when psychological and emotional changes are found to be related to the menstrual cycle, those changes are not viewed within a context of evaluation; as a result, we do not know, for example, whether a statistically significant increase in depression indicates feeling a little sad or clinical depression.

In summary, the widespread belief that a woman's psychological state varies with her menstrual cycle seems to be just that—a belief. Future research, free from the methodological difficulties discussed here, may provide scientific support for this belief, but at this point the evidence is weak. The most that can be said is that there may be a slight trend for women to experience an increase in negative affect during the week prior to their periods and that 6 to 13 days prior to their periods there may be an increased probability that women will die of suicide or disease. The extreme statements that appear in the literature, such as that the premenstruum is "... a time of regression, of an increased libido, poorly controlled by a weakened ego, and of a recurrence of neuroses originally established at the time of puberty" (Tuch, 1975, p. 388) are, perhaps, reflections of cultural stereotypes, rather than conclusions reached through careful evaluation of the empirical research.

Behavioral Covariates
of the Menstrual Cycle

Consistent with the belief that a woman experiences negative affect prior to or during her period is the assumption that a woman's behavior changes and/or her performance deteriorates during the paramenstruum (premenstrual plus menstrual phases). Although the evidence for phase-related negative affect is slight, the assessment of negative affect relies almost exclusively on self-report, and the validity of self-report measures can be questioned on the grounds that they are influenced by response biases, demand characteristics, and belief systems. Task performance and behavior are commonly used, and relatively objective, measures of negative psychological states. For example, learned helplessness, a laboratory analog of reactive depression, is typically assessed by performance on cognitive and instrumental tasks (Seligman, 1975). Consequently, variations in behavior and performance across the menstrual cycle have been the focus of numerous studies.

Table 4.2 presents a summary of 18 studies investigating various aspects of behavior in relation to the menstrual cycle in normal women. The first study did not report statistics, but a description of the data is included. Of the remaining 17 studies, four provided at least some support for the notion that women experience negative behavioral changes or decrements in performance during the paramenstruum. There is evidence for some decrease in arm-hand steadiness and for a greater likelihood of taking one's child to a doctor, of committing crimes of theft and prostitution, and of being involved in an accident during the paramenstruum than during other phases. The last result, that of Dalton (1960b), was true both of active and of passive accidents, the latter being those where another person was responsible and where better judgment on the part of the injured would not have prevented the accident. Three studies reported results opposite to that hypothesized: reaction time and mathematics performance were found to be superior during the luteal phase and to peak premenstrually, cognitive performance was found to be highest during the luteal phase, and women were found to perform better on a practical mechanical test during the paramenstruum than during the intermenstruum. (This last result was one of many analyses done and could have been significant by chance.) Also, estimated time intervals were found to be longest during the premenstruum, but since accuracy was not assessed, it is difficult to interpret these data.

Ten studies in Table 4.2 investigating a wide variety of behaviors, including reaction time, class examinations, and scores on intellectual and mechanical tests, showed no significant variation with phase of the menstrual cycle. Thus, there is little evidence in support of performance decrements occurring during the paramenstruum and considerable evidence to suggest a lack of relationship.

Table 4.2
Studies Relating Behavioral Variables to the Menstrual Cycle

Study	Number of Subjects	Measures	Results
Bernstein (1977)	126	8 course exams during 1 semester.	Compared paramenstrual to intermenstrual. No significant differences.
Dalton (1960a)	217 high-school students	Weekly school grades for 1 term.	Falling marks compared to previous weeks occurred in premenstrual week for 27%, menstrual for 25%, postmenstrual for 10%, intermenstrual for 22%. Rising marks occurred in premenstrual week for 17%, menstrual for 21%, postmenstrual for 30%, intermenstrual for 24%. No statistics reported.
Dalton (1960b)	84	Cycle phase of woman when involved in accident requiring hospitalization.	52% of accidents occurred when women were in paramenstruum. Phase effects significant. True for both active and passive accidents.
Dalton (1961)	156 prisoners	Cycle phase of woman when crime was committed.	Nearly half the crimes were committed during paramenstruum. Phase effects significant. (Crimes were theft and prostitution.)

Study	N	Description	Results
Dor-Shar (1976)	155 replication = 116	Embedded figures test and human figure drawing. Tested once.	Both studies found superior performance in 3rd week (days 14–21). Other weeks similar to one another. No significant results in either study.
Golub (1976a)	50	Cognitive battery tapping sensory-perceptual factors, memory, problem solving, induction, concept formation, creativity. Tested in premenstruum and midcycle.	No significant phase effects.
Graham (1980)	48	Cognitive battery consisting of rod and frame, digit symbol, embedded figures, time estimation, Stroop color-word, porteus maze, addition, and subtraction. Tested once during each phase (follicular, ovulatory, luteal).	Performance significantly better during luteal phase than during follicular and ovulatory phases; this result was due primarily to differences on Stroop and subtraction tests
Hutt, Mychalkiw, & Hughes (1980) Study 1:	12	Choice reaction time tested 4 times per cycle (premenstrual, menstrual, preovulatory, postovulatory) for 2 cycles.	No significant phase effects.
Study 2:	4 (w/premenstrual syndrome)	Choice reaction time tested 3 times per week for 4 weeks.	No significant phase effects.

(continued)

Table 4.2 *(continued)*

Study	Number of Subjects	Measures	Results
Kopell, Lunde, Clayton, & Moos (1969)	8	2-flash threshold, reaction time, time estimation, skin potential. Tested days 3, 14, 24, 26, and 28 for 2 cycles.	Time estimated to be significantly longer in premenstruum than inter-menstruum. No other significant phase effects.
Pierson & Lockhart (1963)	25	Reaction time. Tested days 2, 8, 18, and 26.	No significant phase effects.
Slade & Jenner (1980)	13	Attention task; 2-choice, 4-choice, and 8-choice reaction time task; detection task. Twice a week for 1 cycle.	No significant phase effects.
Sommer (1972)	Study 1: 11 replication = 79	Watson–Glaser Critical Thinking Appraisal. Tested during premen-strual, menstrual, follicular and luteal phases.	No significant phase effects.
	Study 2: 207	Multiple-choice class exams during 1 semester.	No significant phase effects.
Tuch (1975)	140	Length of child's sickness, severity of child's sickness. Cycle phase of mother when she brought child to doctor.	Mothers significantly more likely to bring children to doctor during paramenstruum than during inter-menstruum.

60

Wickham (1958)	Group A: 1,525 taking exam to change job. Group B: 1,000 taking exam to obtain job.	Progressive matrices, mechanical comprehension, arithmetic, squares test, spelling, comprehension, practical mechanics, and verbal. Tested once.	Compared paramenstruum to rest of cycle. Only indication of cycle effect was better performance in paramenstruum on the practical mechanical test for Group B.
Wuttke, Arnold, Becker, Creutzfeldt, Langenstein, & Tirsch (1975)	16	Reaction time, visual orientation, math tasks, memory. Tested every other day for 1 cycle.	Reaction time and math significantly better in luteal than follicular phase with peak 2–4 days prior to menses.
Zimmerman & Parlee (1973)	14	Arm-hand steadiness, GSR to auditory stimuli, reaction time, time estimation, digit-symbol subset of WAIS. Tested during menstrual, follicular, luteal, and premenstrual phases.	Significant differences for arm-hand steadiness: greatest during luteal, lowest during premenstrual. No other significant phase effects.

In an extensive review of the research in this area, Sommer (1973) reached a similar conclusion.

Activity Level
and the Menstrual Cycle:
A New Perspective

The research concerned with physical, psychological, and behavioral covariates of the menstrual cycle has yielded inconsistent and contradictory results. A possible, although at this point speculative, explanation for many contradictory findings might be found by postulating a general increase in activity and/or arousal during the paramenstruum. Altmann, Knowles, and Bull (1941) and Weiner and Elmadjian (1962) observed an increase in physical activity prior to menses; neither study reported statistics, however. Morris and Udry (1970) measured activity in 25 women who wore pedometers for three cycles. Motor activity showed significant peaks on days 2, 15–16, and 27. In addition, Baker and colleagues (1979) found, in three independent samples of women, significantly lower kinesthetic aftereffect scores during the paramenstruum than during the rest of the menstrual cycle; these scores are presumed to reflect stimulus modulation by the central nervous system, and reductions in these scores have been found to be associated with stimulation-seeking behaviors and increased activity levels. Finally, Parlee (1980) found general activation as measured by the Thayer Activation–Deactivation Adjective Check List to be significantly elevated during the premenstrual phase as compared to the remainder of the cycle in seven women studied daily for three cycles.

A paramenstrual increase in physical activity and arousal could account for a variety of paradoxical results in the menstrual cycle literature: (1) Dalton (1960b) found that both passive and active accidents were highest during the paramenstruum; (2) the highest number of stressful events was reported by women in the paramenstrual phase (Wilcoxon, Schrader, and Sherif, 1976); (3) several studies (Kashiwagi, McClure, & Wetzel, 1976; Moos, 1968) have found the premenstruum to be a high point both for both negative and for positive events in the same sample of women; (4) in the review of the literature presented above, the majority of studies found no significant phase effects for selected psychological and behavioral variables; however, of those studies in which significant effects were found, approximately half reported results consistent with the stereotype of negative symptom patterns during the paramenstruum, while the other half reported results in the opposite direction; and, finally, (5) the increases during the premenstruum in the number of crimes committed and in the probability of taking a child to the doctor could simply be due to an increase in activity. In other words, if activity increases, the probability increases that one will engage in any type of activity or have any type of experience.

Others (Koeske, 1980); Parlee, 1980) have postulated similar mechanisms to account for results of their own work on behavioral and psychological changes associated with the menstrual cycle and, in addition, have viewed this hypothesis within the context of a more general theory of emotion. Schacter and Singer (1962) gave subjects injections of epinephrine and then had them observe a stooge modeling either euphoria or anger; subjects uninformed as to the effects of the epinephrine were highly influenced by the stooge and expressed whichever emotion was modeled. The authors concluded that specific emotions are the consequence of an interaction between general arousal and the cognitive interpretation of such arousal. Parlee (1980), whose results were indicative of premenstrual elation rather than premenstrual depression (see Table 4.1), suggested that her subjects were generally healthy and happy women who may have interpreted a premenstrual increase in arousal as evidence of a positive mood state.

In an extension of Schacter and Singer's interactive model of emotion, Koeske (1980) predicted that the cultural stereotype of the premenstrual woman as being depressed and irritable influences which cues, environmental or physiological, are attended to when attaching a label to increased arousal. In her research, subjects were exposed to a variety of situational stimuli consisting of all possible combinations of a premenstrual woman, a nonpremenstrual woman, or a man exhibiting either a positive or a negative mood in a pleasant or unpleasant environment. Subjects attributed negative moods in the premenstrual woman to her biological state but positive moods to her environment. In addition, negative moods in the premenstrual woman were judged as more unreasonable and more indicative of a changeable personality than negative moods in either the nonpremenstrual woman or the man. The author interpreted her data in the context of Schacter and Singer's (1962) interactive theory of emotion; when the woman was described as premenstrual and in a bad mood, the phase of the menstrual cycle was a far more salient cue for the attribution of arousal than were environmental cues, and this may be a reflection of the potency of the stereotypical view of the premenstrual woman. New theoretical perspectives such as the activity/arousal hypothesis presented above and the interactive theory endorsed by Koeske and Parlee offer exciting challenges and prospects for the future of menstrual cycle research.

Conclusions

Considering the minimal empirical support for the belief that the paramenstruum is necessarily a time of psychological and behavioral disaster for women, one must ask how stereotypic beliefs originated and why they are perpetuated. The origins probably date back to primitive societies in which menstruation was viewed as a sign that women were evil, and menstruating women were not allowed to plant, harvest, cook, or associate with men. We are no longer a primitive society; however, according to Delaney, Lupton, and Toth (1977), "Since the advent of modern science, the fears and prejudices surrounding menstruation have given way to an acceptance of it as a normal bodily process—at least in print. But the habits of centuries are not easily unlearned by men who depend on woman's manifest physical differences to give a rationale for their belief in her emotional, economic, and social otherness" (p. 48).

Perpetuation of the stereotype has also been facilitated by the scientific community itself. Parlee (1973) suggested that authors cite past research as support of a theory, without attending to the quality of the cited research. The example she provided is the frequently cited study that claims that there is an association between crashes of women pilots and the phase of their menstrual cycle. The reference is to Whitehead (1934), which ". . . consisted of reports of three airplane crashes over a period of eight months in which the women pilots were said to be menstruating at the time of the crash" (p. 455). Further examples come from frequently cited studies by Dalton. The first (1960c) investigated the relationship between behavioral offenses committed by schoolgirls and their menstrual cycle phase; of a total of 272 offenses during one term, 29% occurred during menstruation. This was a significantly greater percentage than the 14% one would expect to occur by chance during the four days of menstruation, given a 28-day cycle. However, cycle length was not assessed, because, according to Dalton, it varied excessively; thus, the expected percentage of offenses was not accurately calculated, rendering the statistics uninterpretable.

In another study by Dalton (1960a), included in Table 4.2, high-school girls were studied over a period of 12 weeks. During that time, 45% of the girls had only one or two periods, so that almost all of their examinations occurred during weeks labeled as intermenstrual. Furthermore, the primary data were weekly averages of grades, and weeks were labeled rather imprecisely as "premenstrual" if they contained at least three premenstrual days and "menstrual" if they contained at least three menstrual days. Finally, no statistics were reported, so we do not know the probability of these results occurring by chance. In both studies, Dalton concluded that the phase of the menstrual cycle was an important determinant of behavior or performance. Later authors have frequently made general statements referring to these three studies by Dalton and Whitehead as support for deteriorating behavior and performance during the paramenstruum. Thus, one reason for the continued expression of unsupported beliefs is the uncritical acceptance of conclusions from methodologically unsound studies.

Sommer (1973) has suggested that stereotypic beliefs continue because of an editorial bias favoring the publication of studies that find positive results. She states, with reference to menstrual cycle studies, "While the demand for positive results is appropriate when the null hypothesis is assumed, in the case of issues with social implications, often the null hypothesis is not assumed and therefore support may be as important as rejection" (p. 531). Thus, the published research probably reflects only a small portion of the actual research, and the publication of only positive results serves to perpetuate societal attitudes.

The sections above present a review of the literature concerned with physical, psychological, and behavioral variables as they are related to the menstrual cycle in samples of women drawn from a normal population. From the studies reviewed, one must conclude that there is little support for the theory that the menstrual cycle exerts a significant influence on the lives of most women. The intent here is not to minimize the seriousness of menstruation-related disorders; however, the practice of studying menstrual disorders in a normal population maximizes the portion of the variability of the criterion measures due to individual differences. Advantageous utilization of statistical techniques requires that one minimize this source of variability, and one way of accomplishing this is to study samples of women who exhibit a common symptomatology.

The assumption that all women experience menstrual dysfunction not only influences theory, research design, and interpretation, but it may also affect attitudes. Women sufferers and clinicans who view menstrual disorders as being synonymous with being a woman diminish the seriousness with which menstrual disorders are viewed; that is, the attitude that menstrual disorders are a natural part of being a woman suggests that nothing can or should be done to treat the disorders. One effect of such an attitude is noted by Weideger (1976). In a discussion with an endocrinologist as to the benefits of hormone treatment for premenstrual syndrome, the physician responded that ". . . if every woman with premenstrual syndrome went to see an endocrinologist, the physicians would be swamped and unable to offer treatment to anyone else" (p. 54).

II

MENSTRUAL DISORDERS:
DYSMENORRHEA
AND
PREMENSTRUAL SYNDROME

Introduction

Dysmenorrhea and premenstrual syndrome (PMS) are the two most prevalent menstrual disorders, although there is a tremendous range—from 3% (Bickers, 1954) to 100% (Moos, 1968)—in incidence estimates. Although both are generally considered to be psychosomatic disorders, it has been argued that their respective etiologies are strictly psychological (Gregory, 1957) or strictly physiological (Dalton, 1964). The contrasting theoretical orientations derive from several sources. There are both psychological and physical components in the symptomatology; the disorders seem to be exacerbated by stress, which suggests a psychological etiology, yet they covary with distinct hormonal changes, which implies organic causation; and both medical and psychological treatment have been effective to varying degrees. In general, psychological factors tend to be emphasized to a greater degree in theories accounting for PMS than in those accounting for dysmenorrhea. This is undoubtedly due to the fact that "psychological" symptoms, such as depression, comprise the major symptoms of PMS, while "physical" symptoms, such as abdominal pain, are characteristic of dysmenorrhea.

In addition, to the usual problems associated with theoretical conceptualizations and empirical research in the area of psychosomatic medicine—namely, the difficulty of either separating or integrating physiological and psychological factors—the study of PMS and dysmenorrhea has the added burden of having both social and political implications. Women who seek treatment for menstrual disorders are no longer content with ineffective analgesics and advice to stay in bed for a few days each month; they are demanding more effective treatment that will enable them to lead economically independent lives and hold positions of responsibility and influence. These demands, coupled with improved techniques of hormonal assay and a general interest in biorhythms, have precipitated a surge of interest in recent years in the etiology and treatment of PMS and dysmenorrhea.

Symptoms associated with PMS are primarily depression, irritability, lethargy, and water retention, although other symptoms, such as indecisiveness, dizziness, irrationality, constipation, skin disorders, migraine headaches, and graying of hair, have also been mentioned in relation to PMS. Diagnosis generally depends on the idiosyncratic definitions of individual clinicians or researchers, and the presence and severity of symptoms are usually determined by various self-report methods. Structural variables that have been found to be associated with an increased incidence and severity of PMS are age (Dalton, 1964; Moos, 1968), marriage (Coppen & Kessel, 1963), and childbearing (Greene & Dalton, 1953). Individual differences in terms of most salient symptoms, severity of symptoms, and response to treatment are considerable and have led to the speculation that there is more than one distinct disorder under the heading of PMS (Moos, 1969).

The term "dysmenorrhea" is derived from the Greek; it directly translates as painful monthly flow. The present-day medical meaning is painful menstruation, consisting, in general, of cramping and/or pain accompanying the menstrual flow. The discomfort is most intense over the abdomen but may radiate to the thighs and back. Systemic symptoms that occur more infrequently include nausea, vomiting, diarrhea, headache, fatigue, nervousness, and dizziness (Ylikorkala & Dawood, 1978). Although there is considerable individual variability, dysmenorrhea is normally distinguishable from premenstrual syndrome by the type of symptoms and the temporal relationship with the menstrual cycle. The former coincides with the onset of menses and lasts between one and five days, while the latter occurs one to five days prior to, and terminates with, menses. In contrast to PMS, dysmenorrhea has been found to decrease with age and parity (Moos, 1968) and to be unaffected by marriage (Coppen & Kessel, 1963).

The physiological aspects of PMS and dysmenorrhea will be considered separately, as there are distinct bodies of research for each. The literature concerned with psychological and sociocultural factors, however, tends either to not distinguish between the symptoms associated with the two disorders or to combine women with premenstrual symptoms and women with dysmenorrheic symptoms into a single "distressed" group. In addition, the general issues, criticisms, and problems relevant to the psychological and sociocultural literature are similar for both disorders.

5

Psychological Factors
Associated with Dysmenorrhea
and Premenstrual Syndrome

The assumption that personality characteristics, transitory or permanent psychological states, and femininity or acceptance of the
woman's role cause, contribute to, or exacerbate symptoms of menstrual disorders is readily apparent in the literature. This assumption
is manifest in such statements as:

> A consideration of the main syndromes of menstrual distur-
> bance is inseparable from that of the question of the relationship
> between disturbance and neurosis (Gregory, 1957, p. 65).

> Many patients present gynecological symptoms without being
> sick. Their illness represents a psychic conflict sailing under a
> gynecological flag . . . (Rogers, 1950, p. 322).

> If . . . a successful effort is made to modify her attitudes towards
> the acceptance of and pride in her womanly status, then the
> intolerable aspect of her dysmenorrhea, that which brought her
> to the doctor, can be overcome by simple analgesics (Sturgis,
> 1970, p. 150).

One should note that these quotations are from articles published at
least 15 years ago. Since that time there has been a gradual but
perceptible shift away from viewing dysmenorrhea and PMS as
being psychologically caused and toward viewing them as organi-
cally caused. There remains, however, a considerable interest, both

theoretically and empirically, in the psychological correlates of dysmenorrhea and PMS, as is evident in both the professional and popular literature.

Menstrual Disorders and Personality

The vast majority of the research investigating a link between psychological processes and menstrual disorders is of a correlational nature, and the methodology typically consists of measuring menstruation-related symptomatology and personality variables in subjects randomly selected from a normal population. In a large sample of normal college women, Levitt and Lubin (1967) investigated the relationship between frequency and severity of menstrual symptoms and scores on a menstrual attitude survey, the Edwards Personal Preference Schedule, and the Guilford–Zimmerman Temperament Survey. Of 75 correlations performed, 14 were significant and were interpreted to mean that an increased number of menstrual complaints was associated with neurotic and paranoid tendencies and "a set to look at the surface of human behavior." However, such an interpretation should be viewed with caution, since the correlations were small and the means of the personality variables were in the normal range.

In a more recent study, Bloom, Shelton, and Michaels (1978) administered the Menstrual Symptom Questionnaire (MSQ) to 200 women divided into groups that they labeled spasmodic, congestive, and symptom-free. These groups completed the Minnesota Multiphasic Personality Inventory (MMPI), the Personality Research Form, and the Tennessee Self-Concept Scale. In comparison to the symptom-free group, those with spasmodic or congestive disorders scored higher on the depression, psychasthenia, and social introversion scales of the MMPI; on other tests, they scored in the direction of being less autonomous, less prone to play and amusement, less satisfied with themselves, and less positive about their physical and social selves. The authors concluded that, although there were personality differences among the groups, all groups were well within normal limits, and the scores were not indicative of pathology.

Gruba and Rohrbaugh (1975) administered the Menstrual Distress Questionnaire (MDQ) and the MMPI to 60 women. Premen-

strual pain correlated significantly with four MMPI scales, and premenstrual negative affect with two. The MDQ behavior change scale
for symptoms occurring during menses significantly correlated with
two scales of the MMPI. Interpretation of these data is complicated
by the fact that, while pain is characteristic of dysmenorrhea, it is
not typical of PMS; thus, women who complain of premenstrual
pain cannot be classified according to traditional distinctions. Secondly, the authors did not report whether or not the MMPI scale
scores were within normal limits, so we do not know whether
women complaining of menstrual distress were different from
symptom-free women but essentially "normal," or whether they
scored in the pathological range.

Research frequently cited in support of an association between
menstrual symptoms and neuroticism is that by Coppen and Kessel
(1963). A sample of 465 women completed a "menstrual symptom
questionnaire" and the Maudsley Personality Inventory. While dysmenorrhea and neuroticism were not significantly correlated, significant correlations were found between PMS and neuroticism; however, the correlation coefficients ranged between .190 and .297
and thus did not indicate a strong relationship.

Several studies have reported small positive correlations
between degree of menstrual irregularity and the number of symptoms (Moos, 1977; Sheldrake & Cormack, 1976; Wickham, 1958).
Hain and colleagues (1970) found low but significant correlations
between irregularity and some MMPI scales, and comparisons
between extreme groups of irregular and regular women on MMPI
scores yielded significant differences on five of the thirteen scales.
The conclusion of the authors that ". . . regularity of menstrual cycle
. . . is associated with the occurrence of specific and general premenstrual and menstrual symptoms and with personality malad-
justment" (p. 86) seems unwarranted, however, considering that both
groups of women scored within the normal range on the MMPI.

Several researchers have focused on anxiety rather than on
global psychological traits. In one study, pain and cramps during
menstruation, while not related to neuroticism, were found to be
related to anxiety (Hirt, Kurtz, & Ross, 1967). In a later study,
women suffering from PMS scored higher and exhibited more cyclic
variability on the Taylor Manifest Anxiety Scale than did women
who were symptom-free (Halbreich & Kas, 1977). Paige (1973) tested
the hypothesis that anxiety is related to amount of bleeding during
menses. She compared anxiety levels, assessed four times a month

by the Gottschalk–Gleser technique, of women whose flow was reduced due to oral contraceptives and those whose flow remained heavy; women with heavy flow were significantly more anxious than women with light flow.

The research discussed above has frequently been interpreted as supporting the notion that the frequency and/or severity of menstrual symptoms is related to poor adjustment, abnormal personality traits, or neuroticism. A variety of methodological problems in connection with these studies precludes such definitive conclusions. First, in most of these studies, standardized personality tests were employed, and scores on these tests were correlated with measures of menstrual distress. A difficulty in the interpretation of the resulting correlations stems from the fact that similar questions were asked in order to assess both menstrual symptoms and neurotic tendencies. For example, an item on the Maudsley Personality Inventory asks, "Does your mood often go up and down?" Another asks, "Are you sometimes bubbling over with energy and sometimes very sluggish?" On the MMPI we find these items: "Often I can't understand why I have been so cross and grouchy," and "I have periods of such great restlessness that I cannot sit long in a chair." It seems likely that women who would endorse items such as fatigue, restlessness, irritability, or bursts of energy or activity on the MDQ would also answer the MMPI questions in the affirmative.

This criticism is particularly salient when considering that most of these studies do not distinguish between menstrual symptoms that occur only during the paramenstruum and those that occur with equal frequency throughout the menstrual cycle. Clearly, stating that a women experiences premenstrual negative affect is meaningless in terms of menstrual disorders if she experiences negative affect to a similar extent throughout her cycle. One solution to this problem would be to define women as suffering from menstrual distress only if they exhibit significantly more symptoms during the paramenstruum than during the intermenstrual phase. In only one of the studies reviewed here was there a recognition of this problem: in their correlational analyses, Gruba and Rohrbaugh (1975) partialed out the variation in intermenstrual symptom scores. It has been far more common simply to label women as menstrually distressed if they report symptoms during the paramenstruum, regardless of their experiences during the remainder of the cycle. When used in this way, the MDQ and other similar instruments may be measuring general somatic and psychological complaints. Thus, any statistical association noted between scores on menstrual questionnaires and personality scales could be due to the similarity in items and/or a lack of distinction between symptoms occurring during the paramenstruum and those occurring throughout the cycle, rather than to any real association between menstrual disorders and psychopathology.

Additional issues related to methodology preclude a clear interpretation of the results from these studies. The traditional meaning of statistical significance is that a result is significant if it would only occur by chance 5% of the time; therefore, one would expect 5% of independent statistical tests to be significant by chance. In the study by Gruba and Rohrbaugh (1975), 160 correlation coefficients were calculated, of which 16 were statistically significant. Levitt and Lubin (1967) found 14 of 75 to be significant, but, as the authors point out, their computations were not independent, and there is no way to determine chance expectancy with such data. A more serious criticism, perhaps, at least on a theoretical level, is that the large number of coefficients computed in these studies suggests that specific hypotheses are not being tested; the attitude seems to be that if you measure enough variables, something will be significant—and, by chance, something will be. Conclusions from such studies are necessarily tentative.

A related issue concerns the relationship of statistical significance to sample size. As the sample becomes larger, the criterion for significance becomes smaller, so that, for example, in the Levitt and Lubin (1967) study, a correlation coefficient of .18 was significant with a sample size of 221. Statisticians, consequently, advocate reporting R^2 to indicate the degree of association between two variables; R^2 represents the proportion of variance accounted for in one variable by the other variable. Thus, a correlation of .18 represents a relationship in which neuroticism accounts for only 3% of the variance in menstrual distress.

A final criticism of this body of research is related to a rather pervasive theme that the purpose of the research is to confirm "scientifically" the popular belief that women who experience menstrual problems are psychologically ill; this bias manifests itself in some rather unscientific procedures. For example, Hirt, Kurtz, and Ross (1967) correlated scores on the "Semi-objective Criterion for Teenage Dysmenorrhea" with scores from the 16 PF Personality Inventory. The first set of correlations yielded no significant results, so they experimented with different methods of scoring the menstrual questionnaire; in their conclusions, they recommended that the menstrual questionnaire be scored in the manner that produced the highest correlations with the personality scales. A similar bias is evident in the interpretation of the results in a study by Schuckit and colleagues (1974) which compared the frequency of affective symptoms in women with and without PMS. Although the results were in the predicted direction, none of the tests was statistically significant. The authors, however, concluded, "A trend has been found for an association between premenstrual affective syndrome and the occurrence of affective disorder in a population of young women" (p. 517). Although no research is truly objective, in the sense that subjective decisions are necessary concerning the focus, subject population, methodology, analyses, and data interpretation, most researchers make greater attempts at objectivity than that evidenced by these authors.

Several studies that have not relied on a global, correlational approach suggest a small and insignificant contribution of psychological factors in the etiology of menstruation-related disorders. It could be argued that, if PMS symptoms are assciated with the hormonal fluctuations occurring during the cycle rather than with the psychological consequences of menstruation, then PMS symptoms would persist after hysterectomy, since these women are no longer menstruating but continuing to experience the hormonal fluctuations. Beaumont, Richards, and Gelder (1975) found the cyclic variation in mood and physical symptoms to be present, but not significantly so, in women who had undergone a hysterectomy; however, these subjects had not been diagnosed as previously having suffered from PMS. In contrast, Backstrom, Boyle, and Baird (1981) selected seven women undergoing hysterectomy with conservation of the ovaries who had been diagnosed as suffering from PMS. After surgery, cyclical ovarian activity persisted in all subjects, as indicated by changes in excretion of pregnanediol and estrogen. A luteal phase increase in anxiety, tension, irritability, anger, depression, activity, and fatigue persisted after hysterectomy; there was some decrease in feelings of swelling and breast tenderness, but this decrease was not significant. These data argue against a psychological etiology—but are consistent with hormonal etiology—of PMS.

Beard and coworkers (1977) assessed a variety of psychological variables, such as free-floating and phobic anxiety, obsessional traits, depression, AND hysterical symptoms and attitudes, in 18 women complaining of pelvic pain with no abnormality discovered during laparoscopy, in 17 women suffering from pelvic pain with some abnormality that could cause pain, and in 9 women with no gynecological complaints. Women with negative laparoscopy results were significantly more distressed psychologically, according to several variables, than the control group, but they were not significantly different from the women with positive laparoscopy results. In general, the women with evidence of physical abnormality fell between the controls and those with no evidence of physical abnormality on the psychological tests. (Inherent in the authors' interpretation of these data is an assumption of questionable validity—that if a physical abnormality that could account for pain was not discovered during laparoscopy, then a physical cause did not exist.) Both this study and those investigating PMS symptoms after hysterectomy suggest that psychological factors may play a role, but a small and unimpressive one, in the etiology of PMS and dysmenorrhea. Such an interpretation is consistent with the results discussed above of studies correlating menstrual symptoms with personality and psychological variables.

Menstrual Disorders and Femininity

A further psychological variable that has been postulated as being etiological of menstrual symptoms is femininity, or the acceptance of one's role as a woman—the hypothesis being that a woman low on either would resent being a woman and thus would be psychologically susceptible to menstrual disorders. Levitt and Lubin (1967) reported that frequency and severity of menstrual complaints were correlated with a negative attitude toward menstruation. A later study by May (1976) compared women suffering from PMS with women suffering from dysmenorrhea and found the former to feel more resentment over the traditional role expectations (such as that women should be nice, well-behaved, and passively attractive) and more negative about menstruation than the latter group. Berry and McQuire (1972) found a significant association (accounting for 9% of the variance) between the pain, concentration, autonomic reaction, and control scales of the MDQ and low role acceptance.

In contradiction to the results above, which tended toward supporting the hypothesis that menstrual complaints were associated with an unwillingness to accept the traditional feminine role, others have reported significant results suggesting the reverse relationship. Gough (1975) reported small but significant correlations (.15 to .20) between the femininity scale on the California Psychological Inventory and scores on the MDQ, indicating that women who reported more menstrual complaints were more nurturant and deferent and less likely to initiate activity and make decisions than women with fewer menstrual complaints. Consistent with these results are those reported by Paige (1973) who divided her sample according to religious affiliation and noted an association between family and motherhood orientations and menstrual complaints, but only for Catholic women; they were most likely to report symptoms if they believed in motherhood and had no career ambitions.

Similar results have been reported in the most recent of these studies. Chernovetz, Jones, and Hansson (1979) administered the Bem Sex Role Inventory and the MDQ to 84 college women. Femininity scores were significantly and positively correlated with amount of menstrual distress. Surprisingly, women who reported more symptoms signalling the onset of menses had more positive feelings about menses than did symptom-free women; the authors interpreted this last result to mean that reduction of uncertainty as to the time of menses was a greater determinant of feelings than the amount of discomfort experienced. Finally, Woods, Dery, and Most (1982) administered a variety of questionnaires, including a modified MDQ and an instrument assessing attitudes toward menarche, to 193 women. Women with positive recollections of menarche were found to have more severe negative affect and greater performance deficits associated with the paramenstruum than those with negative recollections.

Thus, the data from the studies relating menstrual distress and femininity are somewhat contradictory, and it is difficult to draw any definite conclusions. Furthermore, in postulating role acceptance or femininity as a psychological cause of menstrual disorders, most authors imply that accepting one's role and being feminine are psychologically healthy attitudes. One could, however, logically argue either way—that is, that psychological health is adjusting to one's role, even though it requires being passive and accepting the more dominant social role of men, or that psychological health is rebelling against the inferior role of women in our society.

The Psychological Treatment of Menstrual Disorders

Given the rather extensive research interest in the psychological correlates and etiologies of menstrual disorders, there is surprisingly little research investigating the effectiveness of psychological treatment. In an early study reported by Kroger and Freed (1943), four dysmenorrheic women were treated with the hypnotic suggestion that the next menstrual period would be free from pain and without excessive discomfort. According to the authors, after between 1 and 12 treatment sessions all four were permanently cured. In 1968, Mullen published a case study of a dysmenorrheic woman treated with systematic desensitization in which the imagery was related to the person's behavior before and during menses. The patient was symptom-free after 16 visits. More recently, Tasto and Chesney (1974) treated seven subjects with muscle relaxation paired with imagery associated with menstrual pain reductions, such as a warm bath. The authors reported that there was significant improvement in symptoms but did not indicate whether the women became symptom-free.

Cox (1977) treated 14 menstrually distressed women with systematic densensitization utilizing a menstrual distress hierarchy. According to the Menstrual Symptom Questionnaire (MSQ), seven suffered from congestive disorder (PMS) and seven from spasmodic disorder (dysmenorrhea). There were significant improvements in daily symptom scores, medication usage, and invalid hours, and the treatment was equally effective for spasmodic and congestive disorders. In a more elaborate study, Cox and Meyer (1978) evaluated the effectiveness of systematic desensitization utilizing imagery related to relaxing while anticipating and experiencing the menstrual period. Fourteen distressed subjects, as evaluated by the MSQ, were treated and compared with an equal number of nondistressed subjects on a variety of measures, including severity of symptoms, invalid hours, and number of analgesics consumed. Severity of symptoms was significantly reduced in the treated group but was still significantly higher than in the nondistressed group; at a six-month follow-up assessment the treated group exhibited a continued reduction in symptoms. Again, the treatment was found to be equally successful for spasmodic and congestive disorders. Unfortunately, in none of these studies was there an attempt to control for the reactive effects of monitoring one's symptoms or for the possibility of spontaneous improvement. In order to assess adequately the effectiveness of a particular treatment, the treated subjects need to be compared with a control group who suffer from the same disorder but are not treated, and whose symptoms are assessed in the same way and at the same time.

A no-treatment control group was utilized in a study by Gerrard, Denney, and Basgall (1979), in which dysmenorrheic women were trained in relaxation techniques and then taught to use this training when experiencing menstrual pain. The treated group showed a significant reduction in symptoms compared to the no-treatment control group. In a later study, Quillen and Denney (1982) evaluated a treatment for dysmenorrhea in which the women imagined scenes related to menstrual discomfort; the subjects were then taught to interpret these signs as cues for initiating focal relaxation exercises involving the muscles of the subabdominal area. A total of 24 subjects participated, with 12 in the treatment group and 12 in the control group. All subjects monitored pain, discomfort, interference with life, and amount of time lost for three menstrual cycles. Treated and control subjects did not differ prior to treatment, while after treatment the treated subjects scored significantly lower on all four measures.

Although the last two studies utilized a no-treatment control group, none of the studies included groups with which to evaluate the placebo effects of contact with and attention from a therapist. In order to conclude that improvement was due to the specific treatment utilized, it must be demonstrated that this treatment is superior to "treatment" in which subjects receive attention from a therapist and from which subjects expect to experience improvement. In only one study were placebo effects evaluated. Chesney and Tasto (1975b) divided women suffering from congestive and spasmodic disorders, as assessed by the MSQ, into three groups: one group received treatment in the form of relaxation accompanied by menstruation-related imagery; a second group received pseudo-treatment consisting of discussions on menstruation and home remedies; and a third group was a waiting-list control group. Only women suffering from the spasmodic disorder who received active treatment exhibited improvement (see Figure 5.1). These data suggest that this form of behavior therapy is superior to placebo effects, but only for women suffering from the spasmodic disorder.

There are several difficulties involved with the interpretation of these treatment studies. First, in the three studies that utilized the MSQ to assess symptoms (Cox, 1977; Cox & Meyer, 1978; Chesney & Tasto, 1975b), women suffering from both dysmenorrhea (spasmodic) or PMS (congestive) were treated. However, the symptom checklist utilized to assess improvement consisted of symptoms primarily associated with dysmenorrhea (for example, water retention was not included), and symptoms were assessed only during menstruation, not during the premenstruum. Thus, although the first two studies found improvement for both disorders, PMS or congestive symptoms were not adequately discussed. Second, the most popular psychological treatment for menstrual disorders seems to be some combination of imagery and relaxation. In none of the studies was any attempt made to evaluate the individual contributions of

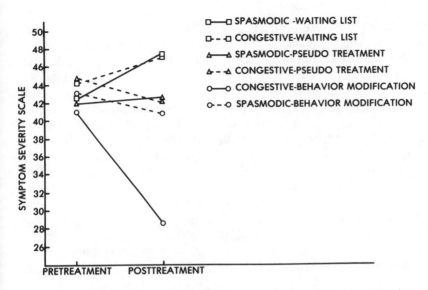

Figure 5.1. Pretreatment and posttreatment group means for menstrual symptoms.

Reprinted by permission From M. A. Chesney and D. L. Tasto, "The effectiveness of behavior modification with spasmodic and congestive dysmenorrhea." *Behavior Research and Therapy,* 1975, *13,* 245–53, Pergamon Press Ltd.

these components of the treatment, so it is unclear whether it was the relaxation or the imagery or the combination that was crucial in effecting improvement.

Issues of Causality

In general, most research investigating a possible psychological etiology for menstrual disorders is correlational, and therefore causality cannot be inferred. Much research can be criticized for at least implying a cause-and-effect relationship from correlational data. A significant association between neuroticism and menstrual symptomatology could mean that neuroticism causes symptoms, that symptoms cause neuroticism, or that a third variable causes both. Despite these limitations on correlational techniques, many investigators suggest a causal link, and one that often reflects experimenter bias. For example, Halbreich and Kas (1977) concluded ". . . women with trait anxiety are predisposed to the PMS" (p. 392), and Levitt and Lubin (1967) suggested that their data ". . . support the gynecologists' contention that an unwholesome attitude toward menstruation may be involved in the etiology of menstrual complaints" (p. 269).

Similarly, it is frequently and erroneously inferred that if a disorder is successfully treated with psychological therapy, then the cause of the disorder is psychological. For example, in the study discussed above by Mullen (1968), the author suggested that his patient's dysmenorrhea was an overt manifestation of her rejection of her femininity. Given that one component of the treatments typically utilized is relaxation, that dysmenorrhea is typically associated with high levels of uterine muscle tension, and that common PMS symptoms are tension and irritability, it is quite possible that the relaxation training simply helps women to reduce general muscle tension, and that this treatment is effective regardless of the original cause.

These interpretational issues are particularly salient when common logic supports either direction of causality, as is the case here. It is equally logical to suppose that, if a woman suffers from regular episodes of pain and depression, which she attributes to menstruation, she then resents being a woman and has a negative attitude toward menstruation or the situation has an effect on her psychological health, as it is to suppose the reverse. On a theoretical level, one can argue a psychological etiology, especially if one considers historical attitudes toward menstruation and the attitudes that are still current today. Primitive societies would not allow women to touch food or associate with men while they were menstruating; present society advertises sanitary napkins with "your secret is safe" and "nothing will show" slogans.

Summary

Although theoretically defensible, a psychological etiology for menstruation-related disorders has yet to be empirically demonstrated. In general, the correlations that support an association between menstrual symptomatology and psychological ill health or lack of role acceptance have been small and account for a minor part of the variability in either variable. Furthermore, the correlational methodology typical of this body of research precludes causal inferences. To establish a causal relationship between menstrual distress and psychological factors, it would be necessary either to manipulate one or both variables or to study the relationship longitudinally. Finally, even in those studies reporting significant correlations, women suffering from menstrual disorders have typically been found to score within normal limits of psychological and personality tests. The continued emphasis on psychogenic theories, despite a lack of empirical evidence, encourages a "blame-the-victim" view of these disorders and diverts attention from demands for improved medical solutions. Lennane and Lennane (1973) commented, with reference to several disorders including dysmenorrhea, that "despite the well-documented presence of organic etiological factors, the therapeutic literature is characterized by an unscientific recourse to psychogenics and a correspondingly inadequate, even derisory, approach to their management" (p. 288).

6

Sociocultural Factors Associated with Dysmenorrhea and Premenstrual Syndrome

There is no doubt that our cultural and societal attitudes and beliefs concerning women and, specifically, menstruation have an impact on menstrual disorders: they affect the reporting of symptoms in both research and clinical settings, the salience of symptoms and their effect on behavior, the likelihood of seeking treatment, the interactions between women patients and gynecologists, and all aspects of research concerned with the investigation of menstrual disorders. In our society, menstruation is generally viewed as a negative event, and the premenstrual and menstrual phases are considered unpleasant times for women. The World Health Organization (1981) conducted a cross-cultural survey on menstruation in 14 countries, on a minimum of 500 women per country. The percentage of women in each country who viewed menstruation as dirty ranged from 7% to 93%; the range of those who viewed it as an illness ranged from 3% to 67%. These cultural differences in attitudes toward menstruation suggest that such attitudes may be determined, to a large extent, by cultural, religious, and historical taboos.

Several studies suggest that attitudes toward menstruation are more negative than is the actual experience of menstruation. Brooks-Gunn and Ruble (1979) compared symptom scores, derived from the Menstrual Distress Questionnaire (MDQ), of premenarchal girls, who completed the form according to what they thought women in general experienced, with scores of postmenarchal girls, who completed the questionnaire according to their own experience; the premenarchal girls expected more severe symptoms than the postmenarchal girls actually experienced. In a later study by the same authors (Brooks-Gunn & Ruble, 1980a), postmenarchal adolescent girls completed the MDQ describing either their own experience or the experience of "girls in general"; subjects describing others had higher scores on the MDQ than subjects describing themselves. Similar differences were found by Golub (1981) when comparing men's descriptions of women's menstrual experiences and women's description of menstrual experiences. Of the men sampled, 75% stated that women's thinking is affected by menstruation, as compared with only 32% of the women. However, the majority of both groups believed women do not function as well and that their personality is different when menstruating.

The apparent importance and variability of attitudes toward menstruation lead Brooks-Gunn and Ruble (1980a) to design the Menstrual Attitude Questionnaire. Items were constructed to include beliefs about physiological and performance concomitants of menstruation, styles of dealing with menses, and general evaluations of menstruation. The original scale consisted of 46 items, and the responses from 191 persons were factor analyzed; 33 items were retained based on the factor structure, and these were cross-validated on an additional 154 subjects. The factors that emerged were labelled as follows: menstruation as a debilitating event; menstruation as a bothersome event; menstruation as a natural event; anticipation and prediction of the onset of menses; and menstruation as having no effect. In general, college women perceived menstruation as natural, somewhat bothersome, and not very debilitating or predictable, while college men perceived menstruation as somewhat debilitating, natural, and bothersome, and quite predictable; both groups agreed that menstruation did have effects.

One would expect that women who perceive menstruation as negative would have more symptoms. In the study by Brooks-Gunn and Ruble (1980a) in which they developed the Menstrual Attitude Questionnaire (MAQ), the MDQ was administered to 191 women. Symptoms reported on the MDQ were not related to the "natural" or "bothersome" scales of the MAQ, but women who perceived menstruation as debilitating and predictable reported more symptoms. Similar results were reported by Woods, Dery, and Ruble (1982), who administered the MAQ and a modified version of the MDQ to 193 women. Care must be exercised in the interpretation of such data—negative attitudes toward menstruation may cause women to perceive symptoms as being more severe than they actually are, and/or experiencing severe symptoms may cause women to develop negative attitudes toward menstruation.

In the cross-cultural study by the World Health Organization (1981) it was found that, in general, those cultural groups in which menstruation was viewed as an illness experienced menstrual discomfort and avoided work outside and inside the home. On the other hand, there was not always a clear, nor necessarily a predictable, relationship between attitudes and symptoms; 93% of Indonesian women and 34% of Korean women viewed menstruation as dirty, while 23% and 52% of these groups, respectively, reported mood changes prior to or during menstruation. Similarly, 61% of Philippino women but only 7% of British women viewed menstruation as an illness, while the majority of both groups—62% and 57%, respectively—reported physical discomfort prior to or during menstruation.

Related to the issue of attitudes and symptoms is a study by Chernovetz, Jones, and Hansson (1979). Both women and men completed the MDQ, with half of each group being ignorant of the menstrual nature of the questionnaire; those men informed as to the menstrual context were told that the purpose of the study was to determine whether symptoms typically related to menstruation also occurred in men. Total MDQ scores were higher for subjects uninformed as to the menstrual context than for those informed, and scores did not differ on the basis of gender. Subjects also rated their general health. For uninformed women, scores on the MDQ and the health ratings were significantly and negatively correlated, while for those women who were informed as to the menstrual context, MDQ scores and health ratings were not significantly correlated. Thus, menstrual and premenstrual discomfort were not viewed as indications of ill health. One could speculate that the reason for this result is the pervasive belief that all women experience menstrual symptoms, and, thus, menstrual symptoms may be viewed as being related more to womanliness than to illness.

There is evidence to suggest that the cultural stereotypic view of menstruation as associated with negative moods and debilitating effects on performance influences causal attributions—attributions being the reasons or causes persons give for their own or others' feelings, behavior, or performance. Koeske and Koeske (1975) had subjects provide attributions for other persons, identified as being premenstrual women, nonpremenstrual women, or men, who were experiencing positive or negative moods in pleasant or unpleasant environments. A clear pattern emerged, in which menstrual cycle attributions were given for negative moods of premenstrual women while other attributions were given for positive moods and for other persons. Campos and Thurow (1978) evaluated attributions provided by women for their self-reported physical and psychological symptoms. The authors hypothesized that women taking birth-control pills would be more likely to make cycle attributions during the premenstrual phase than during other phases because they would be more likely to be aware that they were premenstrual. Consistent with predictions, women on oral contraceptives made more cycle attributions during the premenstrual phase, and women who were medication-free made more cycle attributions during the menstrual phase, suggesting that when menstrual cycle cues are salient, the phase of the cycle is likely to be viewed as causing physical and psychological symptoms.

Historically, a major focus in the attribution literature has been the relationship between attributions and performance (Weiner, 1974). The effects of menstrual cycle attributions on performance were studied by Rodin (1976), whose primary interest was the effects of attributions given for the arousal associated with a task on the performance of that task. In a pilot study, Rodin determined that task attributions ("I am aroused because I am faced with a difficult task") made people fearful and nervous and caused them to perform poorly. Subsequently, she hypothesized that women who attribute high arousal to the phase of their menstrual cycle may perform better than those attributing arousal to the stress inherent in performing a difficult task.

Rodin divided women into high- and low-symptom groups on the basis of the MDQ. After menstrual symptoms had been discussed with the subjects in order to make the cue salient, their performance on cognitive tasks was evaluated under conditions of high arousal (time limit, shocked for poor performance) or low arousal (no time limit, very mild shock) during their menstrual, premenstrual, or intermenstrual phase. Among those tested during the paramenstruum, 16 of 20 high-symptom subjects and 5 of 20 low-symptom subjects attributed their arousal level to the phase of their cycle, while none of the women tested in the midcycle did so. In the high-arousal condition, high-symptom subjects performed significantly better than did low-symptom subjects if tested during the paramenstruum, and similarly to subjects tested in the midcycle; there were no significant performance differences among low-arousal subjects. Thus during the paramenstruum women who experienced symptoms were more likely than women who did not experience symptoms to attribute the arousal associated with a difficult task to their menstrual phase, and this attribution actually seemed to improve their performance. Rodin concluded that high-symptom women do better, either because they are provided with a salient and credible alternative attribution for task-relevant arousal or because they may simply feel that increased effort is required to overcome the debilitating effects of the paramenstruum. This study suggests that, although women may attribute negative events to the phase of their menstrual cycle, such an attribution does not necessarily result in a reduction in performance; indeed, it may even enhance it.

Koeske and Koeske (1975) speculated that menstrual cycle attributions for negative moods may result in self-blame, guilt, and low self-esteem, while Rodin's (1976) data suggest that menstrual cycle attributions for arousal can improve performance. Ruble and Brooks-Gunn (1982) have offered an explanation for this apparent contradiction. The premenstrual and menstrual phases in women who experience menstrual distress may signal a loss of control over emotions or performance, and the literature on the effects of loss of control indicates two possible outcomes: a person may experience reactance, which is operationally defined as the attempt to regain control by increased effort (Brehm, 1972) or learned helplessness, a passive acceptance of the loss of control, indicated by an unwillingness to overcome difficulties and a low self-esteem (Seligman, 1975). Other studies (Gannon, Heiser, & Knight, in press) have reported data to suggest that an individual's response to loss of control, reactance, or learned helplessness is dependent upon one's history—those accustomed to having control are more likely to exhibit reactance—and the degree of uncontrollability—the more uncontrollable the situation, the more likely that learned helplessness will ensue.

Cultural attitudes toward menstruation and menstrual distress are reflected, not only in women's views of their own bodies and experiences, but also in the views of those who treat and research menstrual disorders. Paulson and Wood (1966) developed a 180-item questionnaire consisting of common experiences and feelings and asked eight psychiatrists and eight gynecologists to complete the questionnaire by rating the degree of importance of each item in terms of contributing to a better understanding of dysmenorrhea. Psychiatrists emphasized psychological conflict, early experiences of menstruation, and attitudes toward femininity and womanhood, while the gynecologists viewed the etiology of dysmenorrhea as primarily organic. The results of this study make salient a remark by Kaplan (1964): "It comes as no particular surprise to discover that a scientist formulates problems in a way which requires for their solution just those techniques in which he himself is especially skilled" (p. 31).

In a similar vein, research design and methodology frequently reflect the researchers' biases—the most obvious example being the emphasis on negative events in the study of covariates of the menstrual cycle. Another example reflecting alternative views was pointed out by Sommer (1978): Paige (1971) designed a study to test the hypothesis that heavy menstrual flow may cause women to feel anxious about menstruation, while Peskin (1968) postulated that menstrual flow changed in response to somatization of a psychic conflict. Methodologies determined by the a priori beliefs and the theoretical orientation of the researcher do not necessarily render the research invalid; given the mutually interacting processes that seem to characterize menstrual cycle variables and covariates, both directions of causality are possible, and research designed within the context of either theory could yield potentially valuable information. On the other hand, most investigations of this type are correlational in nature, precluding conclusions pertaining to the direction of causality; and it is in this process of interpretation where researcher bias is frequently and inappropriately manifested by inferring cause-and-effect relationships that accord with prior attitudes and beliefs.

In summary, the research clearly indicates that societal beliefs and stereotypes influence the effects of menstruation and menstrual disorders, both on the behavior and performance of women and on the research on and treatment of menstrual disorders. Of primary interest, however, is the relationship between attitudes toward menstruation and the incidence and severity of menstrual symptoms. Several studies have noted a statistically significant relationship between attitudes and symptoms, but the strength of the association was not impressive and the direction of causality unknown. Furthermore, the World Health Organization's (1981) cross-cultural survey found that the percentage of women in each country who viewed menstruation as "dirty" ranged from 7% to 93%, implying that attitudes toward menstruation are, to a large degree, culture-bound. On the other hand, the incidence of menstrual symptoms exhibited far less variability across cultures; for example, the range of those reporting discomfort associated with menstruation was 50 to 70%. Thus, although attitudes toward menstruation may exert an influence on self-esteem, the likelihood of seeking treatment for menstrual disorders, and men's and women's verbal and behavioral responses to menstrual disorders, they do not appear to account for a major portion of the variability in menstrual symptomatology. According to Weideger (1977), "Painless menstruation or symptom-free menopause are sound goals for medical research, but they ought not to be moral ideals. Perfection of the female spirit will not cure all ills . . ." (p. 243).

7

Physiological Factors
Associated with Dysmenorrhea

There is ample documentation that the direct cause of menstrual cramping and pain is abnormal contractility of the myometrium. Although the early published literature typically did not report standard statistics and significance levels, research over the past 35 years is amazingly consistent in describing the myometrial contractile patterns associated with dysmenorrhea. Contractility during the normal, nonpainful menstrual cycle is characterized by low-amplitude, high-frequency, and somewhat tetanic muscle activity during the follicular phase; during the luteal phase, there is a change to high-amplitude, low-frequency contractions, with reduced tetany; and menses is characterized by similar high-amplitude contractions, with an absence of tetany. Women suffering from dysmenorrhea show similar activity during follicular and luteal phases, but their menses are marked by high-amplitude, irregular or uncoordinated contractions superimposed on a high degree of tetany (Bickers, 1941; Lundstrom, Green, & Wiquist, 1976).

A further difference in myometrial activity between normal and dysmenorrheic women pertains to the differing contractility patterns within the uterus. In the luteal phase, there is a gradient of tonicity between a hypotonic fundus and a hypertonic isthmus, which facilitates retention and implantation of the zygote, should fertilization occur. Immediately prior to menstruation, this gradient is reversed, and the relaxed lower segment allows expulsion of the menstrual product. In painful menstruation, this gradient is frequently such that the isthmus continues to be hypertonic, requiring increased force to expel the uterine lining and blood (Bickers, 1954; Stugis, 1970).

Recordings of myometrial activity during the time when pain is experienced point, once again, to abnormal contractility as the cause of pain. Continuous uterine muscle recordings in dysmenorrheic women demonstrated that periods of high tetany were accompanied by complaints of pain, while the pain dissipated when muscle activity returned to base line between contractions, and that medication that reduced tone also reduced complaints of pain (Filler & Hall, 1970). Akerlund, Andersson, and Ingemarsson (1976) described the pain experienced by their patients as a continuous, dull ache with colicky exacerbations; the continuous component was accompanied by elevated tone, while the colicky component was reported during contractions of high amplitude. Although there is no direct experimental evidence, it is generally believed that this type of muscular activity is painful because the continuously elevated tone produces hypoxia of the uterine muscle (Israel, 1967; Ylikorkala & Dawood, 1978).

Although numerous theories exist to account for dysmenorrhea, and a variety of treatments have been relatively effective, this discussion will be limited to the etiologies and treatments that relate to the most researched areas.

Prostaglandins and the Menstrual Cycle

A current and popular theory concerning the etiology of dysmenorrhea places prostaglandins in a central role. Prostaglandins are a group of biologically active and naturally occurring unsaturated fatty acids with potent actions on blood cells, smooth muscles, fat cells, and nervous tissue. They are found in almost every tissue in the body, particularly in menstrual fluid, the umbilical cord, amniotic fluid, decidua, endometrium, semen, and vesicular glands. Prostaglandins are not stored but are synthesized rapidly, released, and metabolized by the liver, lungs, and alimentary canal (Cooper, Bloom, & Roth, 1982; Speroff & Ramwell, 1970). They are released by cells in response to catecholamines, steroids, inflammation, anaphylaxis, and mechanical stimuli, such as stretching, squeezing, and compression (Sakamoto, Satoh, & Kinoshita, 1976). Prostaglandins are of interest to those concerned with gynecological disorders primarily because they have been hypothesized to be of significant etiological importance in dysmenorrhea. More recently, prostaglandins have also been suggested to be of relevance to other gynecological disorders such as premenstrual tension and endometriosis. Also of interest is that prostaglandins have been investigated as a possible luteolytic factor in humans and animals.

The specific prostaglandins thought to be related to dysmenorrhea are PGE_2 and PGF_{2a}. Several studies have investigated the concentrations of these prostaglandins in endometrial tissue during the normal menstrual cycle. Singh, Baccarini, and Zuspan (1975) measured PGF_{2a} and PGE_2 in endometrial tissue taken during surgery for benign gynecologic disease. PGF_{2a} exhibited little variation during the proliferative phase but markedly increased from the early to the late luteal phase and continued to increase through menses; PGE_2 slightly increased during the luteal phase and then increased dramatically from the late luteal to the menstrual phase (see Figure 7.1). Willman, Collins, and Clayton (1976) have reported

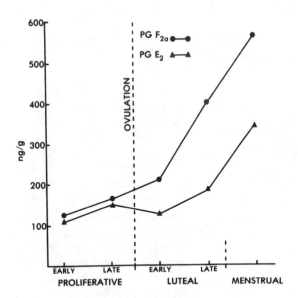

Figure 7.1. Levels of PGF_{2a} and PGE_2 in human endometrium during the menstrual cycle.

Reprinted by permission of the C. V. Mosby Company from E. J. Singh, I. M. Baccarini, and F. P. Zuspan, "Levels of prostaglandins F_{2a} and E_2 in human endometrium during the menstrual cycle." *American Journal of Obstetrics and Gynecology,* 1975, 121, 1003–6.

very similar results, with the levels during menstruation reaching about four times that found during the late secretory phase. Others (Downie, Poyser, & Wunderlich, 1974; Green & Hagenfeldt, 1975) found similar results with a similar methodology. A minor exception is a study by Maathius (1978); in this study, PGF_{2a} increased significantly from early to midluteal phases, consistent with previous studies, but then decreased significantly from the mid- to late luteal phases.

Myometrial prostaglandin concentrations are usually lower than those found in the endometrium, but they apparently also fluctuate with the menstrual cycle. Vijayakumar and Walters (1981) measured PGE_2 and PGF_{2a} and their metabolites in the myometrium of 27 women during abdominal hysterectomy for benign conditions. Throughout most of the cycle, PGE_2 concentrations were greater than PGF_{2a} concentrations; however, this was reversed during the late secretory phase. Myometrial PGE_2 and PGF_{2a} concentrations were highest during the late proliferative phase, and these elevations coincided closely with ovulation. After ovulation, PGE_2 declined, but PGF_{2a} exhibited a second peak during the late secretory phase coinciding with luteolysis and the onset of menstruation.

Researchers have experienced less success in demonstrating variations in prostaglandins in the plasma that could be attributed to the phase of the menstrual cycle. Two studies (Van Orden et al., 1977; Wilks, Wentz, & Jones, 1973) failed to find changes in PGF_{2a} or PGE_2 concentrations in the peripheral plasma during the cycle. Similarly, Jordan and Pokoly (1977) found no fluctuations in prostaglandin concentrations attributable to the phase of the menstrual cycle in either peripheral blood or uterine venous plasma. On the other hand, Aksel, Schomberg, and Hammond (1977) assayed ovarian venous plasma for estrogen, progesterone, and PGF_{2a}. During the luteal phase, the plasma from the active (ovulating) ovary had higher concentrations of PGF_{2a} than did the inactive ovary, whereas there was no difference between the ovaries during the follicular phase. In addition, these authors reported a significant positive relationship between estrogen levels and PGF_{2a} concentrations in plasma from the active ovary during the luteal phase, but no such relationship was found for the inactive ovary nor for either ovary during the follicular phase.

Given that menstrual cycle effects have been demonstrated, at least for endometrial tissue, one could tentatively conclude that prostaglandin production is directly influenced by levels of estrogen and progesterone. Two studies have been designed to investigate the effects of estrogen and progesterone on the production of prostaglandins in vitro. Cane and Villee (1975) have reported that progesterone tended to inhibit PGF_{2a} synthesis while estrogen tended to increase synthesis, although the differences in prostaglandin concentrations between their various cultures did not reach statistical significance. Tsang and Ooi (1982) collected both proliferative and midsecretory endometrial samples and maintained them in cultures with estrogen and/or progesterone and mefenamic acid (a prostaglandin inhibitor). The results on PGF_{2a} are not inconsistent with those above—estrogen increased PGF_{2a} secretion by both proliferative and secretory endometrium; progesterone markedly inhibited PGF_{2a} secretion by proliferative but not secretory endometrium; and neither hormone affected PGE_2. The production of both prostaglandins was inhibited by mefenamic acid. Thus, ovarian hormones may covary with prostaglandin production and may exert a direct causal influence; however, the mechanism by which this occurs remains to be elucidated.

Considerable evidence suggests that prostaglandins have a dramatic effect on the smooth muscle contractions of the vagina, uterus, and ovaries. Of primary interest, again because of the relationship to dysmenorrhea, have been the contractility patterns of the uterus. Two studies (Garrioch, 1978; Hargrove et al., 1976) have found PGF_{2a} to be a potent stimulator of uterine activity; the latter study found PGF_{2a} to have no effect on frequency and amplitude of contractions but to cause a significant increase in tone. Both studies reported that the prostaglandin inhibitor, indomethacin, reduced uterine activity; in the study by Garrioch, the immediate response to the inhibitor was a change to higher amplitude, regular contractions, then diminished tone and amplitude, and, finally, total elimination of spontaneous activity. In 1973, Kirton suggested that the extreme sensitivity of the uterine smooth muscle to prostaglandins supports the hypothesis that prostaglandins act on a specific uterine receptor. Since then, the presence of prostaglandin receptors has been ascertained. Hofmann and colleagues (1983) demonstrated the presence of PGE and PGF_{2a} receptors in the uterus; the highest concentration of receptors was found in the fundus and decreased toward the cervix, and they found a significant correlation between prostaglandin receptors and smooth muscle content of the uterus.

The uterine response to prostaglandins is apparently dependent upon levels of ovarian hormones. Porter and Behrman (1971) examined the influence of progesterone on the myometrial response to PGF_{2a} in the rabbit. The normal uterine response to PGF_{2a} was one of immediate contracture, but in animals pretreated with progesterone the amplitude and duration of the contractions was significantly less than in the untreated animals. Fuchs (1974) tested the uterine response of PGE_1, PGE_2, and PGF_{2a} in rats pretreated with estrogen and/or progesterone. All of the prostaglandins had similar stimulatory effects on contractility, and estrogen tended to diminish the uterine response to prostaglandins, while progesterone enhanced it. Although the results of these studies are contradictory, perhaps because of species differences or variations in methodology, both found the uterine contractile response to prostaglandins to vary as a function of the hormonal environment.

The effects of prostaglandins on other smooth muscle groups have been investigated as well. Coutinho and Darze (1976) assessed the effects of prostaglandins on uterine and cervical contractions. PGF_{2a} was stimulatory in all cases, while PGE_2 relaxed the cervix but stimulated the rest of the uterus, particularly in the preovulatory phase. Ovarian contractility was assessed by Okamura, Okazaki, and Nakajima (1974). Ovarian tissue from 9 of 17 women exhibited a contractile response to PGF_{2a}. However, PGE_1 induced a contractile effect in 5 ovaries and relaxant effect in 4 ovaries of 16 women. Finally, Czekanowski (1975) studied the effects of prostaglandins on vaginal tissue and reported that PGF_{2a} increased contractility, while PGE_1 decreased spontaneous activity. Thus, it is fairly well established that PGF_{2a} is a potent stimulus for smooth muscle activity in much of the reproductive tract; while the data on the effects of PGE are less consistent.

In addition to the effects of prostaglandins on uterine contractility, these substances also appear to have an effect on uterine blood flow. PGF_{2a} has been demonstrated in several studies to be associated with vasoconstriction of the uterine vascular bed (Czekanowski, 1975; McLaughlin, Brennan, & Chez, 1978; Resnik, 1981) while prostaglandins of the E series seem to be potent vasodilators (Clark et al., 1977; Resnik & Brink, 1980). In the study by Clark and coworkers (1977), the administration of a prostaglandin inhibitor reduced PGE levels, increased resistance, and enhanced the vasoconstrictor responses produced by norepinephrine. Schrotenboer and Subark-Sharpe (1981) have speculated that the increases in uterine prostaglandin synthesis just before and during menstruation may cause vasodilation of uterine blood vessels leading to increased menstrual fluid volume, which, in turn, may produce the pain of dysmenorrhea.

It has frequently been hypothesized that degeneration of the corpus luteum in the luteal phase of the menstrual cycle is due to specific luteolytic factors, and PGF_{2a} has been repeatedly hypothesized to be the most likely candidate. PGF_{2a} is luteolytic in most mammals; for example, Sotrel and colleagues (1981) found evidence to support this theory in monkeys. These authors hypothesized that PGF_{2a} causes luteolysis by decreasing the concentration of LH receptors on the corpus luteum, which prevents the corpus luteum from responding adequately to LH, resulting in degeneration.

The luteolytic effect of prostaglandins has been tested repeatedly in humans, and the results have been overwhelmingly consistent and disappointing. The criteria utilized for demonstrating luteolysis have been a decline in levels of progesterone, due to the degenerating corpus luteum, and a shortened luteal phase. Investigations that have administered PGF_{2a} to women at various times during the luteal phase have found neither a decline in progesterone nor a shortened luteal phase (Arrata & Chatterton, 1974; Bolognese & Corson, 1973; Jewelewicz et al., 1972; Wentz, Rocco, & Jones, 1975); others (Coudert, Winter, & Faiman, 1974; Hillier et al., 1972) have found a decline in progesterone levels during infusion of PGF_{2a}; however, upon termination of the infusion, progesterone levels returned to normal, and there was no shortening of the luteal phase. Assuming that exogenously administered prostaglandins exert similar physiological effects as endogenous ones, one can conclude that PGF_{2a} is not a luteolytic agent in women.

Prostaglandins have been demonstrated to influence a variety of biochemical processes in the body. For example, PGE_2 has been found to affect glucose homeostasis by decreasing the metabolism of glucose, decreasing glucose clearance, and inhibiting basal and glucose-stimulated insulin release (Giugliano et al., 1979; Newman & Brodows, 1982). More relevant to the present discussion are several studies presenting evidence for an influence of prostaglandins on LH release. Both PGE_1 and PGF_{2a} have been shown to be effective in stimulating LH release in rats and PGF_{2a} to also increase FSH (Batta, Zanisi, & Martini, 1975; Sato et al., 1974). In a later study (Sato et al., 1975), rats were injected with either PGE_2 or GnRH, and the LH response to both was similar; the authors suggested that the LH response to prostaglandins is mediated by an enhanced GnRH secretion from the hypothalamus.

Other research suggests that prostaglandins have a direct effect on the ovary and facilitate ovulation. Plunkett and colleagues (1975) exposed ovarian tissue to gonadotropins and noted an increase in PGF_{2a} synthesis; these authors hypothesized that prostaglandins cause contraction of the ovarian smooth muscle, which is necessary for follicular rupture. Tsafriri and coworkers (1972) injected rats with indomethacin, a prostaglandin inhibitor; the ovum matured normally, but follicular rupture was prevented. Administering LH to these rats did not overcome the indomethacin block, but administering PGE_2 brought about follicular rupture in most of the rats. Thus, these authors suggested that the antiovulatory action of prostaglandin inhibitors was not due to the blocking of LH release but to a direct action on the follicle.

Although prostaglandins have been shown to have multiple effects on the human body, the mechanism by which these lipids exert their action remains largely a mystery. Newman and Brodows (1982) infused subjects with PGE_2 and noted a significant increase in plasma epinephrine and norepinephrine, which accompanied changes in glucose metabolism and implicates catecholamines in the action of prostaglandins. Giugliano and colleagues (1979) assessed the effects of alpha and beta adrenergic blocking agents, phentolamine and propranolol, on the PGE_1-induced rise in plasma glucose, free fatty acids, glucagon, and growth hormone. The results suggested that the glucagon and free fatty acid responses, but not the glucose and growth hormone responses, were mediated by the beta-adrenergic system.

Czekanowski (1975) noted that both epinephrine and norepinephrine stimulate contractile activity in vaginal tissue in a manner similar to PGF_{2a}, again suggesting that the prostaglandin response may be catecholamine-mediated. On the other hand, Kirton (1973) and Speroff and Ramwell (1970) cite evidence indicating that the prostaglandin effect on uterine contractility is not blocked by atropine, antihistaminic compounds, serotonin antagonists, or alpha or beta adrenergic blockers. Thus, the mechanism by which prostaglandins exert their effects, particularly their effects on the uterus, remains to be clarified.

Dysmenorrhea and Prostaglandins

Currently, the most popular biological theory of dysmenorrhea postulates that dysmenorrheic women have an excessive release of prostaglandins or an excessive sensitivity to their presence. Differences in prostaglandin levels between normal and dysmenorrheic women have been noted. Pulkkinen, Henzl, and Csapo (1978) assessed prostaglandin levels from uterine jet-washings in normal and dysmenorrheic women; the dysmenorrheic women exhibited a greater postovulatory increase in prostaglandins than did the symptom-free women. Data consistent with this have been reported by Lundstrom and Green (1978). They found plasma levels of prostaglandins during menses in normal women to vary between 20 and 33 pg/ml, while those in dysmenorrheic women varied between 32 and 105 pg/ml.

Further evidence for the hypothesized relationship between prostaglandins and dysmenorrhea comes from research studying the effects of the exogenous administration of prostaglandins. Fuchs and Fuchs (1973) reported that the uterine activity resulting from exogenous prostaglandin stimulation was characterized by uncoordinated contractions and an elevation of tone, both of which are properties of uterine activity during painful menstruation. Lundstrom, Green, and Winquist (1976) successfully treated patients with a prostaglandin synthesis inhibitor and then gave one patient an intravenous infusion of PGF_{2a}, which induced severe cramps, a rise in uterine tone, and spastic contractions. Finally, the similarity between the symptoms of dysmenorrhea (flushing, abdominal cramping, nausea, and diarrhea) and the side effects produced by administering prostaglandins to induce abortion and labor has been noted by Halbert and coworkers (1975).

Given the apparent relationships among uterine contractility, prostaglandins, and dysmenorrhea, prostaglandin inhibitors are a logical treatment for dysmenorrhea. A variety of prostaglandin inhibitors are currently available, and they are believed to act by inhibition of over-all prostaglandin synthesis as well as by competition at the prostaglandin receptor site. In studies evaluating the effectiveness of prostaglandin inhibitors on the alleviation of dysmenorrhea, significant or total relief of symptoms has been found for naproxen sodium (Hanson, Izu, & Henzl, 1978; Henzl et al., 1977; Stromberg, Forsling, & Akerlund, 1981), flufenamic acid (Schwartz et al., 1974), ibuprofen (Larkin et al., 1979), and indomethacin (Elder & Kapadia, 1979). One study by Pogmore and Filshie (1980) compared flubiprofen to aspirin and placebo, and no significant differences were found in treatment effectiveness; they ascribed the inconsistency between their results and the overwhelming majority of results from other studies to the fact that flubiprofen inhibits synthesis but, unlike other prostaglandin inhibitors, does not directly antagonize the action of prostaglandins once they are released.

In another series of studies, prostaglandin inhibitors were tested for their effectiveness in treating dysmenorrhea and for their ability to actually inhibit prostaglandin release. Researchers investigating a variety of prostaglandin inhibitors claimed successful treatment effects and found significant reductions in prostaglandin levels in menstrual fluid collected in a cervical cup (Pulkkinen, Henzl, & Csapo, 1978) and from tampons (Chan, Fuchs, & Powell,

1983; Chan, Dawood, & Fuchs, 1979), in uterine jet-washings (Halbert et al., 1975), and in plasma (Rosenwaks et al., 1981). Although, in general, prostaglandin inhibitors afford significant symptomatic relief and significantly reduce prostaglandin levels in groups of women, many individual women are not helped by these drugs. Roy (1983) suggests that one would expect prostaglandin inhibitors to be effective only in women who exhibited an elevated level of prostaglandins. According to Chan, Dawood, and Fuchs (1979), not all dysmenorrheic women do exhibit such high levels; in their sample, those with dysmenorrhea usually had elevated levels of prostaglandins during menses, but two women with dysmenorrhea had normal levels.

In a third series of studies, the treatment effectiveness of prostaglandin inhibitors was determined along with the effects of the drugs on uterine contractility. The results were as follows: Lundstrom, Green, and Winquist (1976) reported symptom relief with indomethacin and a reduced frequency of uterine contractions, as well as greater synchronization of contractions and a reduction in tone; Henzl and coworkers (1979) administered anaprox, which resulted in successful treatment, reductions in uterine tone and amplitude of contractions, and a significant correlation between pain reduction and resting pressure reduction; Smith and Powell (1982) treated dysmenorrheic women with mefenamic acid and found treatment success to be associated with reductions in intrauterine maximum and minimum pressures and with a decreased number of contractions; finally, Csapo, Pulkkinen, and Henzl (1977) found naproxen sodium to be effective in eliminating dysmenorrhea as well as reducing uterine tone and the frequency and amplitude of contractions.

These studies on the treatment effectiveness of prostaglandin inhibitors vary considerably in their methodology: some make no attempt to control for placebo and expectancy effects; others are well designed and compare the effectiveness of prostaglandin inhibitors to analgesics, spasmolytics, and tranquilizing drugs in double-blind cross-over studies and assess effectiveness by a variety of criteria such as pain intensity, interference in daily activities, need for additional analgesics, and general discomfort. Overall, the research provides impressive evidence that prostaglandin inhibitors are an extremely effective method of treating dysmenorrhea and that successful treatment is accompanied by reduced prostaglandin levels as well as reductions in uterine contractility.

The research clearly supports a covarying relationship between the degree of pain accompanying menstruation and endometrial and plasma levels of particular prostaglandins, although the cause of this relationship has not been clarified. Several authors (Downie, Poysen, & Wunderlich, 1974; Halbert et al., 1975; Karim & Hillier, 1973; Schwartz et al., 1974) have suggested that the prostaglandins present in the menstrual fluid originate in the disintegrating endometrium and that, in addition to locally stimulating uterine contractility, they may also be absorbed into the circulation, thereby causing systemic symptoms. Thus, according to this theory, dysmenorrheic women have an excessive release of prostaglandins and, perhaps, an excessive sensitivity to their presence. Others (Filler & Hall, 1970; Lundstrum & Green, 1978; Ylikorkala & Dawood, 1978) have interpreted the elevated prostaglandin levels to be a consequence, rather than a cause, of painful contractions. Cervical obstruction caused either by a small cervical exit or by large fragments of endometrium may increase the contractility required to expel the menstrual product; since prostaglandins are released in response to stretching, the increased muscle contractions may result in increased levels of prostaglandins. Furthermore, a delayed discharge could increase the absorption of protaglandins.

Possibly relevant to resolving the causal nature of the relationship between prostaglandins and dysmenorrhea are data implicating elevated prostaglandin levels with other gynecological disorders. Prostaglandin concentrations above normal have been found in women suffering from endometriosis (Drake et al., 1981; Moon et al., 1981; Willman, Collins, & Clayton, 1976), gynecologic malignancy (Singh et al., 1975; Willman, Collins, & Clayton, 1976), and benign breast disease (Rolland et al., 1979). In addition, prostaglandin inhibitors have been utilized successfully to treat menorrhagia (Anderson et al., 1976) and some symptoms of premenstrual syndrome (Budoff, 1980; Wood & Jakubowicz, 1980). Although research on the relationship between prostaglandins and these disorders has, thus far, been minimal, the available data do suggest that prostaglandins are involved in the biological mechanisms associated with a wide variety of disordered gynecological processes.

Dysmenorrhea
and Vasopressin and Oxytocin

The two hormones of the posterior pituitary, vasopressin and oxytocin, appear to play a role in uterine motility. The primary function of vasopressin (also known as antidiuretic hormone) is to control the rate of water excretion into the urine, and the primary functions of oxytocin are to contract the alveoli of the breasts during nursing and to contract the uterus during delivery. The secretion of both hormones is controlled by nerve fibers originating in the hypothalamus and terminating in the posterior pituitary. Although both hormones stimulate uterine contractility, oxytocin has a lesser effect than does vasopressin on the nonpregnant uterus (Hendricks, 1966).

As with other substances that influence uterine contractility, the effects of oxytocin and vasopressin appear to be dependent upon the levels of ovarian hormones and, therefore, vary with the phase of the menstrual cycle. Hendricks (1966) and Coutinho and Lopes (1968) noted a greater stimulatory effect of vasopressin on uterine motility in the late premenstrual phase and during the first days of menstruation than on other days of the cycle. In the Coutinho and Lopes study, menopausal women treated with estrogen alone exhibited a lack of response to vasopressin throughout the cycle, while those treated with progesterone exhibited a stimulatory response throughout the cycle. Similar results were reported for oxytocin, but, in general, the response to the latter was minimal.

Several investigators have studied the effects on uterine motility of blocking the release of vasopressin. Cobo, Cifuentes, and de Villamizar (1978) blocked vasopressin with a water overload in 27 women during their menses and recorded uterine contractility. There was a decrease in the intensity and frequency of uterine contractions, which was associated with a progressive inhibition of antidiuretic activity. Fuchs and colleagues (1968) recorded intrauterine pressure throughout the menstrual cycle with and without ethanol, which inhibits the release of vasopressin and oxytocin. Spontaneous activity throughout the cycle was similar to that found previously, and the response both to vasopressin and to oxytocin was greatest during menstruation. The inhibitory effect of ethanol was greatest during menstruation, but it did inhibit motility to some extent throughout the cycle. However, both in this study and in an earlier one (Fuchs et al., 1967), it was found that the uterus did respond to exogenous oxytocin and vasopressin during alcohol administration, suggesting that the effect of alcohol is to inhibit release of these hormones from the pituitary rather than having any direct effect on the uterus.

Fuchs (1977) noted that oxytocin seemed to stimulate uterine production of prostaglandins and suggested that prostaglandins mediate the oxytocic reaction. Csapo and Csapo (1974) tested uterine reactivity subsequent to naproxen; PGF_{2a} but not oxytocin restored excitability, which further supports the idea that prostaglandin production is a necessary step in the uterine response to oxytocin. Mechanical dilation of the uterus, cervix, or vagina reflexively stimulates oxytocin release (Hall et al., 1974) suggesting the possibility that cervical obstruction or large endometrial fragments may set off a sequence involving oxytocin and prostaglandin production. On the other hand, there is no direct evidence that dysmenorrheic women have higher levels of oxytocin, greater oxytocin responses, or greater sensitivity to oxytocin than do symptom-free women.

In contrast, others (Akerlund, Stromberg, & Forsling, 1979; Stromberg, Forsling, & Akerlund, 1981) found dysmenorrheic women to have higher concentrations of vasopressin on the first day of the cycle than did women experiencing nonpainful menses. In the latter study, the dysmenorrheic women were compared to symptom-free women on the first day of menses; the dysmenorrheic women were treated with naproxen, which relieved the pain but did not bring down the elevated levels of vasopressin. The authors concluded that elevated vasopressin levels may cause pain by facilitating the release of prostaglandins. In conclusion, the research on oxytocin and vasopressin, as they relate to dysmenorrhea, is sparse; with present knowledge we can only speculate about the roles of these hormones in the development of dysmenorrhea. One might note, however, that a shot of brandy is an old home remedy for menstrual cramps, and alcohol has been found to inhibit the release of oxytocin and vasopressin.

Dysmenorrhea
and the Autonomic Nervous System

The smooth muscle of the uterus is innervated by the sympathetic nervous system, although the type of innervation differs morphologically and functionally from other types of sympathetic nerves (Pulkkinen, 1970). While the postganglionic fibers of most sympathetic nerves synapse near the spinal cord and, thus, extend from the spinal cord to the target organ, those that innervate the uterus synapse in a variety of locations—some very close to myometrial cells (Moawad, 1973). The myometrium contains both alpha and beta adrenergic receptors and is, therefore, responsive to both epinephrine and norepinephrine.

Sullivan and Marshall (1970) exposed isolated myometrial strips to a variety of neurotransmitters and blocking agents. These in vitro preparations responded to norepinephrine with increased motility in a dose-related manner. The tissue was also tested under the influence of an alpha blocker (phentolamine) and a beta blocker (propranolol); the alpha blocker inhibited the norepinephrine-induced stimulation, while the beta blocker had a slight excitatory effect, suggesting that norepinephrine acts on the myometrium via alpha receptors. In addition, Moawad (1973) cites further evidence to suggest that epinephrine causes inhibition of uterine motility and that this inhibition is mediated via beta receptors. Supporting evidence has been reported by Lehrer (1965), who found that stimulation of alpha receptors caused an increase in tone, while stimulation of beta receptors had little effect unless high concentrations of stimulants were used, and then a fall in tone was observed.

Given that uterine motility exhibits consistent patterns during the menstrual cycle and that these patterns vary with the phase of the cycle, it is not surprising that researchers have concluded that the ovarian hormones influence uterine motility—specifically, that progesterone is inhibitory and estrogen stimulatory (Gibor et al., 1971; Raz, Zeigler, & Adoni, 1971; Sweat & Bryson, 1970). Furthermore, there is evidence to suggest that estrogen and progesterone exhibit such effects through their actions on myometrial alpha and beta receptors (Sporrong et al., 1977). Research by Akerlund and Andersson (1976) and Cibils (1971) indicates that the natural variability in estrogen and progesterone throughout the menstrual cycle is responsible for the fluctuating receptivity of the adrenergic receptors. In the former study (Akerlund & Andersson, 1976) terbutaline, a beta-receptor stimulator, was found to exert its strongest effects during the secretory phase of the cycle, and this was thought to be due to an increased sensitivity to beta-receptor stimulation brought about by high levels of progesterone.

Raz, Zeigler, and Adoni (1971) pretreated rats with a variety of combinations of hormones and receptor blockers, then tested the effects of epinephrine on the motility of isolated myometrial strips. In general, epinephrine, which stimulates beta receptors, exhibited an inhibitory effect on motility, and this effect was enhanced by progesterone and blocked by propanolol. Bottari and coworkers (1983) assessed alpha-1 and alpha-2 receptor content in myometrial tissue obtained from premenopausal women in different phases of the menstrual cycle, postmenopausal women, women at term pregnancy, and those receiving progesterone treatment. The affinity and number of alpha-1 receptors were similar in all conditions, whereas the number of alpha-2 adrenergic receptors increased concomitantly with plasma estradiol levels. Furthermore, the increase, apparently due to estrogen, was counteracted by progesterone. These studies are fairly consistent in indicating that alpha-receptor stimulation increases uterine motility, beta-receptor stimulation decreases motility, and estrogen enhances either the number of or the sensitivity to alpha receptors, while progesterone has similar effects on beta receptors. Thus, uterine motility appears to be a reflection of the interactions among the quantity and sensitivity of myometrial alpha and beta receptors, the hormonal environment, plasma levels of epinephrine and norepinephrine, and the activity of the sympathetic nervous system.

The autonomic nervous system innervates not only the uterine smooth muscle but also the vasculature that supplies blood to this muscle. Since a possible source of the pain in dysmenorrhea is hypoxia of the uterine muscle, it is possible that vasodilation would increase blood flow and relieve the pain associated with uterine muscle activity and, conversely, that vasoconstriction of these arterioles would exacerbate the pain. The research concerned with the innervation of the uterine blood supply has indicated that vasodilation is effected via beta receptors (Akerlund & Anderson, 1976; Greiss, 1972) and that vasoconstriction is effected via alpha receptors (Dyer & Gough, 1971; Gough & Dyer, 1971). In the study by Greiss, castrated ewes were pretreated with estrogen, alone or with progesterone, and the differing hormonal environments were found to have no effect on the uterine vasculature response to adrenergic stimulation. On the other hand, estrogen and progesterone do appear to influence uterine blood flow (see discussion below), but the response to these hormones does not seem to be mediated by the autonomic nervous system (Resnik et al., 1976).

The assumption that beta receptors mediate a relaxation effect on the myometrium and vasodilation of the uterine vasculature has provided the rationale for the development of experimental treatment programs for women with dysmenorrhea. Hansen and Secher (1975) tested a beta-receptor-stimulating drug on 47 women with dysmenorrhea in a double-blind study. The drug provided symptomatic relief for only 10 women, and 25 of the 47 had unpleasant side effects such as palpitations and quivering. Akerlund, Andersson, and Ingemarsson (1976) gave 11 dysmenorrheic women terbutaline, which is a selective beta-receptor agonist. In addition to monitoring subjective reports of pain, the authors monitored uterine motility. In all the women the drug reduced pain and either totally or partially inhibited myometrial activity. In two studies (Csapo, Pitkanen, & Pulkkinen, 1975; Nesheim & Walloe, 1976), the beta-receptor stimulator, isoxsuprine, was evaluated for its treatment effectiveness in dysmenorrhea. The latter study found no significant improvement, while the former found the drug to cause a significant reduction in uterine contractility and pain. In most of these studies, significant negative side effects were noted which precludes the use of beta-receptor stimulators for widespread treatment of dysmenorrhea. However, these studies do provide data that increase our understanding of the mechanisms of uterine motility.

Dysmenorrhea and Estrogen and Progesterone

A general belief is apparent in the literature that dysmenorrhea is the result of an excess of progesterone or a high progesterone-estrogen ratio in the late luteal phase of the menstrual cycle. Ylikorkala and Dawood (1978) suggested that, since dysmenorrhea occurs only in ovulatory cycles, a secretory endometrium and progesterone are necessary preprequisites for dysmenorrhea. Dalton (1964) has agreed with this theory and has reported that women whom she has treated for premenstrual tension with progesterone injections have occasionally developed dysmenorrhea. On the other hand, as Israel (1967) has pointed out, neither an estrogen/progesterone imbalance nor an excess of progesterone has been demonstrated in the blood or urine of women suffering from dysmenorrhea.

More research has been done in this area since Israel's conclusion. Ylikorkala, Puolakka, and Kauppila (1979) compared hormonal levels in dysmenorrheic and normal women; progesterone levels and the progesterone–estrogen ratio did not differ among the two groups, but the dysmenorrheic women had significantly higher levels of estrogen late in the cycle than did the normal women. In a similar study, Akerlund and colleagues (1979) found dysmenorrheic women and women experiencing nonpainful menstruation to have similar levels of progesterone and estrogen but only assessed hormone levels on Day 1 of the cycle. In a final study of this type, Webster (1980) assessed a variety of symptoms related to premenstrual tension and dysmenorrhea and plasma levels of estrogen, progesterone, testosterone, LH, FSH, and prolactin at 13 points during the menstrual cycle; the resulting correlations between symptoms and hormones revealed no significant relationships between menstrual cramps and estrogen, progesterone, or the ratio of the two. Thus, there is little direct evidence to suggest that plasma levels of estrogen or progesterone are potentially important in the etiology of dysmenorrhea.

On the other hand, there is considerable indirect evidence that links the ovarian hormones to dysmenorrhea. It is well known that the administration of estrogen and progesterone in the form of oral contraceptives tends to relieve dysmenorrhea (e.g., Bickers, 1954; Israel, 1967; Sheldrake & Cormack, 1976). The uterine motility during anovulatory cycles is characterized by hypotonia, and labor-like patterns are absent; and it has been assumed that this reduced uterine motility results from the absence of a progesterone-producing corpus luteum (Sturgis, 1970). In marked contrast are results reported by Cullberg (1972). He studied the effects on dysmenorrhea of different oral contraceptives containing various amounts of progesterone; dysmenorrhea was relieved by progesterone-dominated compounds in a dose-related manner.

A number of other theories have been advanced to explain why oral contraceptives, or anovulation due to some other cause, tends to diminish the symptoms of dysmenorrhea. It has been suggested that oral contraceptives reduce myometrial contractility by directly reducing the levels of prostaglandins (Ylikorkala & Dawood, 1978), that oral contraceptives reduce prostaglandin levels by preventing a secretory endometrium (Sturgis & Albright, 1940), and that there is less menstrual product in anovulatory cycles, so there is less uterine contractility required to expel it (Bickers, 1954). Another possibility is that estrogen and progesterone influence dysmenorrhea indirectly by modifying other variables associated with contractility. In the discussion above, evidence was presented to suggest that estrogen tended to increase endometrial levels of PGF_{2a}, while progesterone had the opposite effect, that estrogen diminished and progesterone enhanced the uterine response to vasopressin, and that the uterine response to prostaglandins varied with levels of estrogen and progesterone, although not in a consistent manner.

A further possibility is that estrogen and progesterone levels may influence uterine blood flow and, in this way, exacerbate or relieve the hypoxia associated with exaggerated uterine contractility. Exogenous estrogen has been found to cause dilation of the uterine vasculature, and the degree of vasodilation has been found to be inversely proportional to progesterone levels (Anderson & Hackshaw, 1974; Resnik, 1981). Greiss and Anderson (1970) reported that exogenous estrogen increased uterine blood flow, that exogenous progesterone alone had little effect, and that progesterone administered after daily estrogen caused about a 30% decrease in uterine blood flow in castrated ewes. The mechanism by which the ovarian hormones affect uterine blood flow has not been clarified, although Resnik and coworkers (1976) have suggested that the dilation response to estrogen is not mediated by the autonomic nervous system, since their research indicated that neither propanolol nor atropine blocked the response.

Summary

The research clearly indicates that dysmenorrhea is associated with uterine motility characterized by high-amplitude, asychronous, or uncoordinated contractions superimposed on an elevated tone, that such motility patterns are accompanied by elevated levels of prostaglandins, that women who suffer from dysmenorrhea exhibit higher levels of prostaglandins than those experiencing painless menstruation, and that prostaglandin inhibitors are an effective treatment for dysmenorrhea. Although these results have been found to be true for the vast majority of women tested, a small minority who experience dysmenorrhea do not exhibit elevated prostaglandin levels and/or are not successfully treated with prostaglandin inhibitors. Still open to question is the cause of the elevated prostaglandin levels. The hypothesized mechanisms by which the synthesis and release of prostaglandins are enchanced include elevated levels of vasopressin or oxytocin and abnormal levels of estrogen or progesterone. As yet, there is only minimal empirical support for the role of any of these hormones as being etiological in dysmenorrhea.

Since prostaglandins are released from tissue in response to squeezing or stretching, elevated levels of prostaglandins in dysmenorrheic women may be a response to cramping rather than the cause of it. The successful treatment of dysmenorrhea with prostaglandin inhibitors weakens this argument but does not entirely negate it. It is possible, for example, that cramping increases prostaglandin synthesis and release, which, in turn, increases cramping, and so on in a mutually interacting fashion and that prostaglandin inhibitors interrupt this spiraling effect. If dysmenorrhea is initiated by increased uterine motility and simply exacerbated by the resulting release of prostaglandins, we are still left with the question of what is the cause of the initial cramping.

One possibility is that cervical obstruction due either to a small cervical exit or to large fragments of endometrium may require greater levels of contractility to expel the menstrual product. A second possibility is that the increased contractility is caused by increased alpha receptor stimulation by the autonomic nervous system and/or by increased levels of plasma catecholamines; either or both would enhance motility and favor vasoconstriction of the arterioles supplying blood to the uterine muscle. Autonomic nervous system activity and plasma catecholamine levels are influenced by a wide variety of factors—one being psychological stress. Thus, levels of anxiety, environmental stressors, or fear, for example, may be causally related to dysmenorrhea. Research on psychological factors, such as anxiety and fear, has not been supportive of such an interpretation; however, as was pointed out in a preceding section, the methodological inadequacies that characterize this body of research preclude definitive inferences. The relationship between environmental stress and dysmenorrhea is yet to be studied.

8

Physiological Factors Associated with Premenstrual Syndrome

Premenstrual Syndrome and Estrogen and Progesterone

Because PMS occurs a a time in the menstrual cycle when progesterone is normally at its peak, most theories that posit a physiological etiology for PMS attribute the symptoms either directly or indirectly to progesterone. Some suggest that women suffering from PMS produce too much progesterone, others that they produce too little; some say that the estrogen–progesterone ratio is too high or too low, and still others that although the absolute quantities of progesterone and estrogen may be normal, women who suffer from PMS have an abnormal physiological response to one or both of the hormones.

The most common theoretical orientation among researchers and clinicians concerned with PMS is that this disorder is caused by an insufficiency of progesterone or an insufficiency of progesterone relative to estrogen—that is, a high estrogen–progesterone ratio. This theory was originally derived from speculation based on clinical observations by Dalton (1964) who noted that women who suffer from PMS either have a worsening of symptoms or a complete relief of symptoms during pregnancy, which she attributes, respectively, to a lower-than-normal or normal production of progesterone from the placenta. Others (e.g., Hackmann, Wirz-Justice, & Lichtsteiner, 1973) have noted the similarity in symptoms occurring during the premenstruum, the postpartum period, and the menopause—all of

110

which are accompanied by a rapid decline in progesterone. Anzalone (1977) assessed a number of physiological, psychological, and sociological variables in terms of their ability to predict which women would suffer from postpartum depression; the best predictor was a history of PMS. Such observations have led some to suspect that the factor responsible for the symptoms associated with these events may be genetically determined abnormality in progesterone metabolism (Hamburg, 1966).

Considering the prevalence of the assumption that PMS results from abnormal hormonal levels, there are surprisingly little direct data to offer as support for such a theory. Webster (1980) assessed hormonal levels and symptoms throughout two menstrual cycles in 37 women; none of the typical PMS symptoms were significantly correlated to estrogen, progesterone, or some ratio of the two hormones. Her sample was, however, a random one and not selected on the basis of the presence or absence of PMS, so it is difficult to generalize from this sample to women who suffer from PMS. Morton (1950) measured hormonal levels in 29 psychiatric patients who complained of premenstrual symptoms; 26 had a relative excess of estrogen compared to progesterone, but the author did not compare these levels with those of a symptom-free group.

A more adequate methodology for assessing the hormonal hypothesis of PMS requires that subjects who suffer from PMS symptoms be carefully selected and compared to symptom-free women. Smith (1975) compared hormonal levels of women suffering from premenstrual depression with those of women who were symptom-free. Mean levels of plasma progesterone were lower for patients than for controls, while estrogen levels and estrogen–progesterone ratios did not differ between groups. [The relationships between hormonal levels and symptoms in a group of women suffering from slight to moderate PMS was studied by Backstrom and Mattsson (1975). High correlations, ranging from .453 to .720, were reported between estrogen levels and estrogen–progesterone ratios and feelings of anxiety, irritability, and depression; there were no significant correlations between progesterone and any symptom.]

In a methodologically somewhat more sophisticated study, Dennerstein and coworkers (1983) evaluated 30 women with complaints of severe premenstrual tension and 89 women without premenstrual complaints. Subjects rated symptoms daily on a 10-point scale and collected 12-hour overnight urine specimens daily for one menstrual cycle. The urine samples were assayed for estrogen and pregnanediol, an end-product of progesterone metabolism.

Significantly lower pregnanediol values were found in the PMS patients throughout the cycle when compared with those from the symptom-free controls. In further analyses, utilizing data from only those subjects who complained of premenstrual symptoms, the authors correlated ovarian steroids and symptoms and found no significant correlations. However, recognizing that a time lag may occur between fluctuations in hormones and resulting symptoms, they employed auto-correlation techniques to determine the time lag representing maximal concordance between the variables. Pregnanediol was not correlated with symptoms at any time lag; however, estrogen exhibited maximum concordance and significant correlations with irritability and swelling with a time delay of seven days. These data suggest that high levels of estrogen are associated with increased symptom severity and that the symptoms follow the elevated estrogen levels by about a week.

The widespread use of oral contraceptives during the last 15 years has provided a readily available population of women who have artificially altered hormonal levels, and the results of studies with such samples may be informative in determining the effects of exogenous hormones on symptoms associated with PMS. Kutner and Brown (1972) studied psychological symptoms in women who had never used oral contraceptives, in those who were past users, and in current users. Current users reported significantly less premenstrual moodiness and irritability than the other two groups, and users of combination-type pills reported less of both symptoms than sequential-type users. Within the group of combination-pill users, those who were taking pills with a high progesterone content experienced less depression than those taking pills with little progesterone. Similar results were reported by Paige (1971), whose subjects taking combination-type oral contraceptives experienced less phasic fluctuation in anxiety and hostility than subjects not taking oral contraceptives. Similar improvement was not effected through use of sequential-type pills. These studies offer indirect evidence for reduced symptomatology being associated with increased levels of progesterone.

In contrast, Grant and Pryse-Davies (1968), in a large sample studied longitudinally, compared the incidence of depression and endometrial monoamine oxidase (MAO) levels among women taking a wide variety of oral contraceptives. The use of strongly progestogenic, combination-type pills was associated with elevated levels of endometrial MAO and a high (28%) incidence of depression, while strongly estrogenic, sequential-type pills were associated with lowered levels of MAO and a low (7%) incidence of depression.

Cullberg (1972) tested three types of oral contraceptives—with high, moderate, and low progesterone content, with estrogen content held constant. Approximately one-third of each group suffered adverse mental changes in response to the medication. Further analyses were done by breaking down the groups into those with and those without a history of premenstrual irritability; subjects who reacted negatively to high progestogenic compounds were mainly those who did not previously suffer from premenstrual irritability, while those subjects who reacted negatively to high estrogenic compounds were mainly those with a history of premenstrual irritability. These results agree with Dalton's research and support the "low progesterone" or "high unopposed estrogen" theory of PMS. These results also serve to emphasize the necessity of studying PMS in women who experience PMS rather than in the general population.

The contradictions evident in the research on the effect of oral contraceptives on PMS symptoms are obvious but may be, at least partially, explained by the confounding of a general psychological state and transitory psychological distress occurring during the premenstruum. Only in the study by Kutner and Brown (1972) were symptoms specific to the premenstrual period evaluated in relation to the effects of oral contraceptives; in the other studies, general affect throughout the menstrual cycle was assessed. It is certainly possible that the exacerbation or alleviation of symptoms occurring premenstrually and the modifications of general affect could be influenced via different mechanisms.

The Premenstrual Migraine

One PMS symptom that has received individual attention is the premenstrual migraine. Although migraine headaches are often included in listings of PMS symptoms, they are not experienced by all women who suffer from PMS. Kudrow (1978) has proposed a theoretical model outlining the biochemical changes that culminate in a migraine attack. According to his theory, high levels of serotonin cause the cerebrovascular constriction that is responsible for the prodomal phase of the headache; this is followed by serotonin depletion, which allows for an unopposed vasodilation, contributing to the painful phase of the migraine. Kudrow suggests that the initial increase in serotonin is caused by platelet aggregation, which can be induced by a variety of factors, one of which is increased levels of estrogen. Therefore, according to this theory, high levels of estrogen may precipitate a headache.

The empirical support for Kudrow's or any theory relating ovarian hormones to migraine is inconsistent and inconclusive. Epstein, Hockaday, and Hockaday (1975) collected blood daily throughout one menstrual cycle from eight women with menstrually related migraine, six with migraine that was not related to menstruation, and eight headache-free controls. Mean plasma estrogen and progesterone levels were significantly higher in migraine patients than in controls for most of the cycle, with the largest differences being in progesterone during the late luteal phase. However, there were no significant hormonal differences between women whose migraine was related to cycle phase and those whose migraine occurred at random with respect to the menstrual cycle. Furthermore, "No specific hormone changes were associated with the occurrence of a migraine attack, nor did rising or falling levels, or greater increments of change over given cycle phases, appear important in provoking attacks" (p. 543).

Somerville (1971) investigated the hypothesis that the premenstrual migraine is precipitated by the natural fall of progesterone in the late luteal phase. He collected daily blood samples from women who suffered from migraine headaches that were clearly related to their menstrual cycle as well as from women who were headache-free. Half of the women with migraines were treated with progesterone injected daily, beginning three to six days prior to the expected onset of menses. There were no significant differences in progesterone levels between untreated migraine patients and the controls. All of the untreated migraine patients developed a premenstrual headache—one at the onset of the falling phase of progesterone, one during this phase, and three at its termination. Four of the five treated patients experienced their usual premenstrual headache, and the chacteristics of these headaches were similar to those experienced prior to medication. The author concluded that progesterone withdrawal does not seem to be the cause of the premenstrual migraine.

Since progesterone did not seem to be the culprit in premenstrual migraines, Somerville (1975) then investigated the hypothesis that estrogen withdrawal is responsible for this symptom. He first tried to prevent a migraine in four women suffering from premenstrual migraine by administering either an injection of estrogen, which raised plasma levels, over several days or oral estrogen to produce a short peak in estrogen; neither treatment was effective, and all four patients had a migraine. In the next cycle, these women were given oral estrogen beginning five to six days before the expected menses, and the estrogen was continued until the patient got a headache or until menses ceased. Three of the four women experienced a migraine at the usual time. In four other patients, after they had experienced their usual migraine, they were given a long-acting estrogen injection, which caused a fairly sustained elevation in plasma estrogen levels. This artificially produced surge of estrogen resulted, in two of these subjects, in a typical migraine at the end of the estrogen withdrawal; in one an atypical migraine occurred, and one experienced no headache. Somerville interpreted these data to mean that estrogen withdrawal after a period of sustained elevation may precipitate a migraine attack. Although Somerville's data offer more support for an estrogenic mechanism in causing premenstrual migraines than for a progesteronic one, the evidence is not impressive, and the role of ovarian hormones in the etiology of migraine remains to be elucidated.

Premenstrual Depression

Perhaps the most commonly experienced symptom among women suffering from PMS is depression. It has been noted among clinicians that depression is a frequent complaint, not only of PMS sufferers, but also of menopausal women and of women taking oral contraceptives. Since oral contraceptives produce an abnormal hormonal environment, menopause is associated with substantial changes in hormonal status, and the premenstruum is characterized by falling levels of estrogen and progesterone, it is reasonable to hypothesize an hormonal etiology for premenstrual depression. In a previous chapter, the research concerned with mood fluctuations that covary with the menstrual cycle in symptom-free women was reviewed. It was concluded that, although there may be a slight trend toward negative affect premenstrually, normal hormonal fluctuations cannot account for the degree of depressive affect reported by PMS sufferers. However, premenstrual depression could be due to abnormalities in the levels of estrogen or progesterone, in the ratio of the two, or in the biologic sensitivity to estrogen or progesterone.

MAO has been postulated as the mediating mechanism responsible for the empirical relationship between hormones and depression. One theory of endogenous depression is that an excess of MAO reduces available norepinephrine, resulting in slowed or reduced central neural activity. Evidence for this theory is primarily indirect and stems from the ability of MAO inhibitors to effect clinical improvement in depression. (It should be pointed out that all of the studies discussed in this section measured either plasma MAO or endometrial MAO, while the theory being evaluated refers to brain MAO; and endometrial and/or systemic MAO levels do not necessarily reflect levels in the central nervous system.)

Several studies have found higher levels of MAO in the secretory endometrium than in the proliferative endometrium (Grant & Pryse-Davies, 1968; Southgate et al., 1968). Gilmore and colleagues (1971) failed to find menstrual cycle phase effects in plasma or platelet MAO and concluded that the previously found fluctuations were local to specific organs rather than systemic. On the other hand, significant increases in plasma MAO from the follicular to the luteal phase were reported by Klaiber and coworkers (1971). A later study (Klaiber et al., 1972), comparing normal and endogenously depressed women, showed depressed women having significantly higher levels of plasma MAO than normal women. Both groups exhibited higher MAO levels during the luteal phase than during the follicular phase, and this difference was significant for the normals but not for the depressed women.

The research above indicates that depression is associated with elevated levels of MAO and that MAO is, in general, higher in the luteal phase than in the follicular phase. Since estrogen is high in both the follicular and the luteal phases, and progesterone is present, in quantity, only in the luteal phase, one might logically infer that progesterone is, in some way, implicated in the differential MAO levels. Nevertheless, the available research suggests that a lack of estrogen is responsible for elevated levels of MAO. Exogenous estrogen has been found to reduce elevated MAO levels in endogenously depressed women and to be significantly better than placebo in reducing MAO levels and depressive affect in women hospitalized for depression (Klaiber et al., 1972). In the latter study, neither the absolute level of MAO nor the change in MAO was significantly correlated with depression, so other factors may be involved.

Research on the influence of oral contraceptives on PMS symptoms is discussed above. Of the three studies that specifically assessed depression, data from two implied that the progesterone component of the pill was related to alleviation of depression (Kutner & Brown, 1972; Cullberg, 1972), while one suggested that progesterone exacerbated depression (Grant & Pryse-Davies, 1968). Several studies have found the oral-contraceptive-induced depression to be relieved by pyridoxine (vitamin B6) therapy (Baumblatt & Winston, 1970; Adams et al., 1973). In the latter study, the oral contraceptive varied in progesterone content and the amount of progesterone seemed unrelated to depression. Adams and colleagues (1973) have speculated as to the specific mechanism involved in the depression and the apparent relief afforded by pyridoxine. These authors suggested that the estrogen component of the oral contraceptives is responsible for the depression in that estrogen increases cortisol activity in the liver, and hydrocortisone administration greatly increases hepatic tryptophan oxygenase levels, which, in turn, increase the requirements of vitamin B6 to achieve normal production of serotonin. Thus, without vitamin B6 supplements, exogenous estrogen causes a reduction in brain serotonin, which may be associated with depression.

It is difficult to integrate results and draw conclusions from studies that vary considerably in methodologies. One would expect that the relationship between hormones and mood will vary with the subject population—PMS sufferers, clinically depressed, or symptom-free persons—and with whether the hormonal states are endogenous or are altered artificially. Furthermore, the primary weakness of this body of research is the lack of studies utilizing samples of PMS sufferers.

Given these limitations, the research results and their interpretations presented here are rather consistent in suggesting that hormones, both endogenous and exogenous, can modify mood. Contradictions exist, however, as to which of the hormones—estrogen or progesterone—is responsible for the observed effects. MAO fluctuations associated with the menstrual cycles of symptom-free women and the beneficial effects of exogenous estrogen on MAO levels and affect in clinically depressed women implicate a low estrogen–progesterone ratio as being associated with depression. In contrast, the proposed theoretical explanation for contraceptive-induced depression and its alleviation with pyridoxine indicts the estrogen component of the pill as being responsible for the depression. It is, of course, possible that the cause of depression varies among individuals—one woman may experience premenstrual depression due to an exaggerated increase in MAO during the luteal phase, perhaps as a result of inadequate levels of estrogen, while another woman's depression may be caused by luteal-phase reductions in serotonin associated with unusually high levels of estrogen or a high estrogen–progesterone ratio.

Hormonal Treatment of PMS

Several studies have assessed the treatment effectiveness on PMS of exogenous progesterone. Dalton (1964) viewed PMS essentially as a disorder resulting from lower-than-normal levels of progesterone and claimed overwhelming success in alleviating symptoms with progesterone therapy. In a clinical report of 78 patients (Greene & Dalton, 1953), women suffering from severe PMS were treated either with intramuscular progesterone injections or with implants; 83.5% became symptom-free from injections, 6.6% improved, and 6.6% reported no relief. Women suffering from mild or moderate PMS were treated with ethisterone, a synthetic progesterone that may be taken orally; 47.9% reported complete relief and 17.4% partial relief. Of the 14 patients who did not improve, 9 experienced complete relief with progesterone injections.

Aware of the inconvenience and expense of regular injections, Dalton (1959a) tested the effects of three oral progestogens on PMS symptoms in 58 patients who had experienced complete relief of symptoms from progesterone injections. Good or moderate relief was reported by 59% who received ethisterone, 37% who received dimesthisterone, and 59% who received norethisterone. Similar results were reported by Rees (1953), who treated 30 patients suffering from severe PMS. In the five patients treated with intramuscular injections of progesterone, PMS symptoms were alleviated. All 30 patients were treated with ethisterone for some cycles, and in 85% of the trials "significant" (no statistics were reported) relief was obtained. No relief was noted during cycles in which placebo tablets were administered. Dalton (1964) speculated that while both forms (oral and injected) of treatment affect the endometrium in a similar way, only injected progesterone provides a sodium-dissipating action, which accounts for its greater treatment effectiveness.

In a group of 30 women with moderate or severe PMS, Appleby

(1960) compared the treatment effectiveness of meprobamate (a tranquilizer), chlorothiazide (a diuretic), and oral progesterone and noted total or marked relief of symptoms in one-half, one-third, and one-fifth of the patients, respectively. The author commented that rarely did a patient respond to more than one form of treatment, suggesting multiple etiologies and optimal treatments for PMS. In another study, which compared the effectiveness of various drugs, Ylostalo and colleagues (1982) treated 36 women suffering from PMS. All patients received placebos during the first and fourth cycle and either bromocriptine or norethisterone during the second and third cycle; 11 out of 17 preferred bromocriptine over the placebo, and 12 out of 19 preferred norethisterone over placebo. For the symptoms of breast engorgement, edema, irritability, and depression, bromocriptine was found to be effective by 67 to 96% of the patients, norethisterone by 72 to 100%, and placebo by 33 to 57%. Bromocriptine was significantly more effective than placebo for breast engorgement, irritability, and depression, while norethisterone was significantly more effective than placebo only for breast engorgement.

This last study makes salient the importance of comparing treatments to a placebo when evaluating their effectiveness. The vast majority of research that has attempted to evaluate the treatment effectiveness of progesterone has failed to do this, and, although progesterone is becoming increasingly popular as a treatment, empirical validation is lacking. Furthermore, as Reid and Yen (1983) have pointed out, most women who suffer from PMS exhibit normal levels of progesterone. However, they conclude that ". . . the doses of progesterone recommended by Dalton are, in most cases, much greater than those needed to achieve normal luteal phase progesterone levels. . . . It remains possible, therefore, that pharmacologic doses of progesterone may have some unknown central effects that could explain the apparent amelioration of PMS" (p. 711).

Summary

Dalton's (1964) hormonal theory of PMS hypothesizes that PMS symptoms are caused by insufficient progesterone, excess estrogen, or excess estrogen relative to progesterone in the late luteal phase of the menstrual cycle. The few studies in which women suffering from PMS have been compared to symptom-free women on levels of estrogen and progesterone offer empirical validation for this theory.

In contrast, studies that have focused on specific symptoms, such as migraine headache and depression, have been less supportive of a hormonal etiology of PMS. In the case of depression, levels of estrogen and/or progesterone have been found to modify mood, and MAO levels tend to covary with the menstrual cycle; although such results are relevant and provocative, research utilizing subjects who suffer from PMS is noticeably absent. Perhaps most damaging to this theory are the data on the treatment effectiveness of progesterone. Although progesterone has been found to be a moderately successful treatment, it has not been demonstrated to be more effective than diuretics, tranquilizers, or placebos.

PMS and Fluid Retention

Common complaints among women suffering from PMS are weight gain, swelling, and a bloated feeling prior to menstruation, suggesting a common etiology of exaggerated fluid retention premenstrually. Currently, the primary mechanisms accounting for fluid retention as being the cause of some PMS symptoms are thought to be related to the renin–angiotensin–aldosterone system and to prolactin—both of which have known influences on sodium, potassium, and water retention and excretion.

The variability in substances that relate to water retention throughout the menstrual cycle has been the focus of several studies. Janowsky, Berens, and Davis (1973) reported an increase during the luteal phase in the urinary potassium–sodium ratio which peaked three days prior to menses and decreased on the first day of bleeding. Voda (1980) studied biochemical indicators of edema in 24 women by collecting blood and urine every other day for one cycle. Serum sodium levels did not increase premenstrually, while serum potassium levels increased above base line in the luteal phase and dropped at the end of the luteal phase. In contrast, Gray and coworkers (1968) found no phase effects of potassium–sodium ratio, and Michelakis, Stant, and Brill (1971) found no significant change in exchangeable sodium space that could be attributed to the menstrual cycle. Others have measured weight as an indicator of fluid retention. Andersch and colleagues (1978) and Voda (1980) failed to find weight to covary with the cycle, while Janowsky, Berens, and Davis (1973) found a significant correlation (.47) between weight and potassium–sodium ratio. Weight variation was also reported by Abramson and Torghele (1961), who noted menstrual, midcycle, and premenstrual peaks. Similarly, an average weight fluctuation of .7 lbs was reported for 69 subjects by Golub, Menduke, and Conly (1965), but the subjects differed as to where in the cycle they weighed the most. Thus, in samples of women not selected on the basis of PMS complaints, there seems to be little evidence that fluid, weight, or the related electrolytes vary as a function of the phase of the menstrual cycle.

Perhaps more relevant to a discussion on PMS is research in which fluid and electrolytes were assessed in women who suffer from PMS. Andersch and colleagues (1978) measured total body water, total potassium, and weight in women suffering from PMS and in women who were symptom-free. PMS women experienced more variability in body water and had more body water per mol of body potassium in the luteal phase than did the controls; however, body water was not higher during the luteal phase than during the follicular phase. Although the results were somewhat inconsistent, the authors concluded that PMS symptoms are accompanied by changes in fluid retention; since weight did not vary, the authors suggested that these changes are a function of a redistribution of fluid rather than an absolute increase.

Further evidence comes from Wong and coworkers (1972), who measured the capillary filtration coefficient (CFC) as an index of the integrity of the vessel wall to water. Women with symptoms of PMS showed clear cyclic fluctuations, with CFC increasing throughout the cycle and peaking just prior to menstruation, while control women without PMS showed a relatively constant CFC throughout the cycle. On the other hand, Herzberg (1971) assessed electrolytes premenstrually and at another point in the cycle in 11 women suffering from severe premenstrual tension. He found no significant differences among cycle phases in total exchangeable sodium, extracellular sodium, residual sodium, intracellular water, or extracellular water but did find total body water to be significantly decreased premenstrually. Thus, research investigating changes in parameters associated with water retention as a function of menstrual cycle phase in normal women or as a function of the presence or absence of PMS symptoms has been somewhat supportive of fluid retention increasing premenstrually, but the considerable variability in methodology and results that characterizes this research renders integration and interpretation difficult.

Another method of assessing the impact of water retention on PMS is to evaluate the treatment effectiveness of diuretics. Appleby (1960) treated 30 women suffering from PMS with chlorothiazide, approximately one-third of whom reported total or marked relief of symptoms. In another study, ammonium chloride was found to be effective in preventing swelling but did not always relieve tension, irritability, depression, or anxiety (Rees, 1953). Singer, Cheng, and Schou (1974) tested the effectiveness of lithium in a treatment based on its diuretic action in addition to lithium's known effects on periodic psychiatric disorders. Patients improved with both lithium and placebo, and although lithium was better at relieving symptoms, the differences were not significant. Lithium, chlorthalidone, and a placebo were compared on their effectiveness in treating PMS in a study by Mattsson and Schoultz (1974). The placebo was preferred by most patients. However, those who responded well to lithium had pronounced premenstrual weight increases prior to treatment but not during treatment. Thus, the treatment effectiveness of diuretics is variable, although there is some support for their use, especially for women whose primary symptoms are those of swelling, heaviness, weight increase, and bloating.

The Renin–Angiotensin–Aldosterone Hypothesis

Aldosterone has been implicated as an etiological agent in the fluid and electrolyte changes that may be responsible for some PMS symptoms. Aldosterone is the primary mineralocorticoid secreted by the adrenal cortex, and its main function is to regulate electrolyte balance, especially that of sodium and potassium. The regulation of aldosterone release begins in the hypothalamus, which secretes corticotropin-releasing hormone into the portal system supplying the anterior pituitary. The anterior pituitary, in response, releases adrenocorticotropic hormone (ACTH). ACTH plays a permissive role in the release of aldosterone in that it allows the primary regulatory factors, potassium and angiotensin, to act directly on the adrenal cortex.

The hormone angiotensin II is one of the most potent vasoconstrictors known. When blood flow through the kidneys decreases, the juxtaglomerular cells secrete renin into the blood, where it acts to form angiotensin I. Angiotensin I then circulates to the lungs, where it is converted to angiotensin II. A major effect of angiotensin II is to cause arteriole, and to a lesser extent venule, vasoconstriction. Angiotensin also acts on the kidneys to decrease salt and water excretion, and it causes the release of aldosterone from the adrenal cortex. Aldosterone, in turn, causes sodium to be retained in the extracellular fluid and potassium to be excreted in the urine. Due to the increases in sodium retention, water reabsorption and retention occurs as well. Thus, aldosterone can cause a dramatic increase in the extracellular fluid volume. In addition to these effects, blood volume and cardiac output are also increased. A brief excess of aldosterone is accompanied by compensatory changes to reduce blood pressure; however, prolonged elevations of aldosterone may cause moderate or severe hypertension.

Because of the effects of the renin–angiotensin–aldosterone system on water retention, which is viewed as a possible contributor to PMS, there has been an interest in studying the effects of the ovarian hormones on this system and in determining the variability in these substances accounted for by menstrual cycle phase. Studies assessing levels of these substances during the menstrual cycle have yielded the following results: (1) three of four subjects showed phasic changes during the menstrual cycle in plasma renin activity and plasma aldosterone, although the phase of peak activity varied among the subjects (Katz & Romfh, 1972); (2) in six subjects, the average level of plasma renin and plasma aldosterone was twice as high in the luteal phase than in the follicular phase, with peak activity occurring around days 22–25 (Michelakis, Yoshida, & Dormois, 1975); (3) aldosterone was significantly higher during the second half of the cycle than during the first half (Brown et al., 1964; Gray et al., 1968; Schwartz & Abraham, 1975); (4) plasma renin and renin concentration increased significantly during the luteal phase in six subjects (Skinner, Lumbers, & Symonds, 1969); (5) plasma angiotensin II and aldosterone increased from the early follicular phase to the late luteal phase (Sundsfjord & Aakvaag, 1970).

From such data, one would expect that as aldosterone levels increased in the luteal phase, there would be a concomitant increase in potassium–sodium ratio, water retention, and weight; however, as discussed above, such results have not been consistently found. Furthermore, Voda (1980) measured aldosterone, weight, serum, and urinary sodium and potassium, as well as psychological and somatic symptoms, in 24 women during one complete cycle. Aldosterone was not significantly correlated with weight, sodium, potassium, or any of the psychological or somatic symptoms. It should be noted, however, that these studies utilized samples of normal women—a sample selected on the basis of PMS complaints may have yielded differing results, since women with PMS may have abnormal levels of aldosterone or an abnormal sensitivity or response to normal levels.

Despite the lack of empirical support for the role of aldosterone in the etiology of PMS, O'Brien and colleagues (1979) evaluated the effectiveness of spironolactone, an aldosterone antagonist, in the treatment of PMS. A sample of 28 included women both with and without symptoms of PMS. Blood samples and mood assessment were taken repeatedly throughout four cycles in a double-blind cross-over trial of the drug. Although spironolactone was associated with a noticeable decrease in symptoms, there were no significant correlations between symptoms and premenstrual aldosterone levels. Interestingly, prior to the administration of the drug, women with PMS symptoms exhibited lower aldosterone levels than women without symptoms, although this difference was not significant.

Although direct evidence implicating aldosterone in the etiology of PMS is lacking, studies have consistently found a higher level of aldosterone, renin, and angiotensin in the luteal phase of the menstrual cycle than in the follicular phase, and it has been suggested that progesterone is the causal agent of this luteal phase elevation. In the study by Voda (1980), significant correlations were found between progesterone and aldosterone throughout the menstrual cycle (see Figure 8.1). Michelakis and coworkers (1975) reported that the typical increases in renin and aldosterone noted in the luteal phase did not occur in anovulatory cycles—again suggesting a role for progesterone in promoting aldosterone secretion. Two studies (Laidlaw, Ruse, & Gornall, 1962; Landau & Lugibihl, 1958) administered exogenous progesterone and assessed the resulting effects on sodium excretion. Their data suggest that progesterone is a natriuretic agent in that it causes initial sodium diuresis followed by a rebound period of sodium retention. Sundsfjord and Aakvaag (1970) advanced the hypothesis that a direct action of progesterone is to promote diuresis through sodium excretion; the decreased sodium levels then stimulate an increased production of renin and angiotensin II, which, in turn, stimulates the adrenal cortex to release aldosterone. In other words, the increased levels of renin and aldosterone may not lead to changes in water volume and metabolites because these substances are being produced in order to counteract the sodium-excreting property of progesterone and, thus, restore a homeostatic state.

A different method of inquiry into the relationship between sex hormones and the renin–angiotensin–aldosterone system has been to assess the effects of oral contraceptives on this system. Unfortunately, this has not been done in a systematic manner, and the resulting data are somewhat contradictory. In general, oral

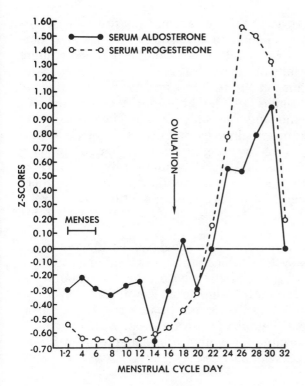

Figure 8.1. Pattern of aldosterone and progesterone over a 32-day period. (Values represent z-score variable transformation of raw data, each data point representing the number of variable transformed units above or below the mean of 0.)

From Ann Voda, "Pattern of progesterone and aldosterone in ovulating women during the menstrual cycle." In Alice J. Dan, Effie A. Graham, and Carol P. Beecher (Eds.), *The Menstrual Cycle, Volume 1: A Synthesis of Interdisciplinary Research,* p. 230. Copyright © 1980 by the University of Illinois. Published by Springer Publishing Company, Inc., New York, Used by permission of the publisher.

contraceptives tend to increase levels of renin, angiotensin, and aldosterone, although these effects may be absent or reversed, depending upon whether the subject remains normotensive or develops hypertension as a result of the treatment (Tapia, Johnson, & Strong, 1973). The oral contraceptives utilized in these studies contained both estrogen and progesterone compounds, but researchers have suggested that it is the estrogen component that was responsible for the changes in this system and any resultant hypertensive effects. Estrogen is known to have sodium-retaining properties and, thus, could be responsible for an increase in blood volume and, ultimately, hypertension (Laragh, 1976).

Further information on the role of estrogen was reported by Nowaczynski and colleagues (1978), who studied the effects of oral contraceptives on bound and free aldosterone. They found that although total aldosterone remained essentially unchanged, the percentage of bound aldosterone was significantly higher and the percentage of free lower in those taking oral contraceptives than in the medication-free controls. Of interest was their finding that there seemed to be a physiological dose–response relationship between the estrogen content of the oral contraceptives and the level of this binding.

In summary, hypothesizing abnormalities in the renin–angiotensin–aldosterone system to account for particular symptoms of PMS is appealing in light of the phase differences found for aldosterone and its covariation with ovarian steroids. However, the diverse and contradictory results cannot be integrated in a meaningful way at this point. Perhaps future research, which tests this hypothesis directly by evaluating women who suffer from PMS, will yield more rewarding answers.

The Prolactin Hypothesis

Prolactin is a hormone secreted by the anterior pituitary. Dopaminergic neurons in the hypothalamus synthesize prolactin inhibitory factor (PIF), which is transmitted to the anterior pituitary where it effects continuous inhibition of prolactin secretion. Elevated levels of prolactin during the luteal phase of the menstrual cycle have been implicated as causal in those symptoms of PMS associated with fluid retention. The reasoning behind this hypothesis is that progesterone tends to inhibit the secretion of prolactin (Halbreich et al., 1976), and prolactin facilitates the retention of sodium, potassium, and water (Andersch et al., 1978). Thus, lower-than-normal levels of progesterone could act to increase prolactin and, thus, increase fluid and electrolyte retention.

Prolactin fluctuations during the normal menstrual cycle have been the focus of several studies. Both Ehara and colleagues (1973) and Aksel (1981) reported no phase differences in plasma prolactin. On the other hand, Maslar and Riddick (1979) measured tissue content and in vitro production of prolactin of endometrial samples;

no prolactin was detected in the tissue or the medium in endometrial samples obtained prior to cycle day 22. However, total prolactin in tissue and medium increased significantly between cycle days 22–24 and days 25–26. The authors concluded that prolactin is synthesized by the endometrium and that the degree of synthesis corresponds to the deciduation of the stroma.

Of obvious interest to the prolactin hypothesis are those studies that have looked for elevated levels of prolactin in women suffering from PMS. Halbreich and coworkers (1976) measured serum prolactin levels during the menstrual cycle in women with and without PMS. Throughout the cycle, women suffering from PMS had significantly higher levels of prolactin and greater increases during the premenstruum than did the controls. On the other hand, two recent studies (Backstrum & Aakvaag, 1981; O'Brien & Symonds, 1982) examined plasma prolactin levels in women with and without PMS, and neither study found significant or consistent differences in prolactin between the two groups. In addition, Mason (1975) has pointed out that increases in prolactin may occur in response to psychological stress, so the direction of causality in the relationship between prolactin and symptoms in women with PMS would not be obvious if such a relationship were, indeed, found.

Despite the lack of evidence linking prolactin and PMS, treatments based on such a relationship have been evaluated. Bromocriptine is a long-acting dopamine receptor agonist and, as such, increases the action of hypothalamic neurons that synthesize prolactin inhibitory factor; bromocriptine thus inhibits the release of prolactin by increasing central nervous system inhibition of its release. Research on bromocriptine has validated this drug as a prolactin suppressant by demonstrating significant reductions in prolactin during treatment (Andersen et al., 1977). On the other hand, bromocriptine has been found to have no effect on body weight or total body water (Andersch et al., 1978).

In evaluating bromocriptine as a treatment for PMS, Ghose and Coppen (1977) found it to be no more effective than a placebo in reducing subjective symptoms. Others have been more successful in demonstrating treatment effectiveness. Andersen and colleagues (1977) found breast tenderness, but not other symptoms, to be significantly better with bromocriptine than with placebo. Benedek-Jaszmann and Hearn-Sturtevant (1976) compared bromocriptine and a placebo in a double-blind crossover study. Women treated with the drug experienced significant improvement in breast symptoms, edema, weight gain, and mood; the placebo afforded no similar improvement. Elsner and coworkers (1980) found only breast symptoms to be significantly better with bromocriptine than with placebo, while Ylostalo and colleagues (1982) found bromocriptine to be significantly better than placebo for both breast tenderness and irritability.

To summarize, although prolactin may facilitate the retention of water, sodium, and potassium and, therefore, be a likely candidate to investigate as an etiological agent in PMS, the empirical evidence offers little support for such a hypothesis. Women suffering from PMS have not consistently been found to have elevated levels of prolactin, and suppression of prolactin release from the anterior pituitary seems to be useful in alleviating some symptoms, particularly breast tenderness, but it offers little relief for other symptoms associated with PMS.

PMS and Carbohydrate Metabolism

Carbohydrate metabolism is potentially relevant to the study of PMS because hypoglycemia, or low blood sugar, is characterized by a variety of symptoms similar to those described by women who suffer from PMS, such as fatigue, anxiety, excitation, and depression. Dalton (1964) included hypoglycemia as one of many premenstrual symptoms.

Surprisingly few studies have evaluated carbohydrate metabolism in women with PMS. In an early study, Morton (1950) examined 20 psychiatric patients who reported premenstrual symptoms; 16 of them showed signs of hypoglycemia as measured by a glucose tolerance test, and the timing of the hypoglycemia corresponded to the self-report of symptoms. In a later study by Morton and coworkers (1965), half of a group of 249 women prisoners suffering from PMS were given a combined treatment of a diuretic, an antispasmodic, a mild stimulant, vitamin B, and a supplementary protein diet; 79% of the women reported improvement in symptoms. Unfortunately, only 12 women were given a glucose tolerance test, which revealed a pronounced hypoglycemic reaction. Posttreatment tests showed these subjects exhibiting less reaction, but they still had lower-than-normal blood sugar. In neither study were statistics reported or control groups included, and the latter study was not designed to separate the effects of various treatments.

Smith and Sauder (1969) investigated the popular belief that women crave sweets, particularly chocolate, prior to their menstrual period. In a pilot study they interviewed 37 psychiatric inpatients or patients recently released whose primary diagnosis was depression; of these patients, women who also reported PMS were significantly more likely to also report a craving for sweets and chocolate than those without PMS symptoms. They than gave a questionnaire to 289 nurses to assess their eating habits and symptoms associated with PMS. Those who reported premenstrual feelings of tension or depression were more likely to report compulsive eating and cravings for sweets than non-PMS women, but not necessarily during the premenstrual week. Such data are of some interest, but not only is the reliability and validity of the data questionable because of its retrospective nature, but there is no evidence that such cravings are related to hypoglycemia. Indeed, one argument opposed to a hypoglycemic explanation of PMS is that PMS does not seem to be relieved by the ingestion of food (Reid & Yen, 1981).

Under normal conditions, carbohydrate metabolism is regulated by several interacting systems. The hypothalamic–pituitary–adrenal system is responsible for the production of cortisol. Cortisol, a glucocorticoid, stimulates gluconeogenesis, the formation of glucose from amino acids and glycerol, and decreases the rate of glucose utilization by cells. Both of these processes would tend to increase blood sugar levels. Regulation of cortisol levels begins in the hypothalamus, which secretes corticotropin-releasing hormone (CRH) into the portal system that supplies the anterior pituitary. The anterior pituitary, thus stimulated, releases adrenocorticotropin hormone (ACTH) which acts on the adrenal cortex to release glucocorticoids, about 95% of which is in the form of cortisol. Cortisol exerts a negative feedback effect at the level both of the hypothalamus and of the anterior pituitary; when cortisol reaches high levels, it inhibits the release of hypothalamic CRH and pituitary ACTH. This feedback system operates effectively to maintain optimal levels of cortisol under nonstressful conditions, during which times cortisol production is almost entirely dependent upon ACTH-initiated stimulation of the adrenal cortex. However, this inhibitory feedback can be readily overcome by stress, which is a powerful stimulus for the release of CRH and, ultimately, cortisol. Thus, physical or psychological stress causes an immediate and marked increase in CRH, ACTH, and, within minutes, cortisol.

Other regulatory mechanisms of carbohydrate metabolism include insulin, probably the major regulator of blood sugar levels, which is secreted by the pancreas and causes uptake, storage, and utilization of glucose—the result of which is to decrease blood sugar levels. Insulin is released in response to high circulating levels of glucose. Growth hormone, a product of the anterior pituitary, also affects the carbohydrate metabolism and does so by decreasing glucose utilization by the cells, enhancing glycogen deposition, and decreasing the uptake of glucose by the cells—the general effect being to increase blood sugar levels.

A common method for assessing carbohydrate metabolism is the glucose tolerance test. This test provides an assessment of the body's ability to metabolize carbohydrates and is based on the fact that oral intake of glucose stimulates insulin release by the pancreas. A load of glucose is administered and glucose is measured in the blood and/or urine. Test results revealing either elevated or diminished blood glucose are indicative of abnormality; diabetes is suspected with elevated blood glucose levels.

Relevant to the hypothesis relating hypoglycemia to PMS is the body of research that has studied the effects of endogenous and exogenous estrogen and progesterone on carbohydrate metabolism. The effects of endogenous hormones have been evaluated by assessing changes in measures of carbohydrate metabolism throughout the menstrual cycle. Genazzani and colleagues (1975) found growth hormone to decrease significantly during the luteal phase of the menstrual cycle; and two studies (de Pirro et al., 1978; Bertoli et al., 1980) have reported lower insulin binding during the luteal phase than during the follicular phase. Since growth hormone tends to increase blood sugar levels and since less insulin binding would result in greater levels of biologically active insulin, results from both studies suggest possible mechanisms for lowered blood sugar during the luteal phase of the menstrual cycle.

Other studies have examined the influence of menstrual cycle phase on blood cortisol levels. Beck and coworkers (1972) reported significant decreases in cortisol during the luteal phase compared with the proliferative phase; cortisol was measured twice during the cycle, on days 10 and 24. On the other hand, two more recent studies (Carr et al., 1979; Parker et al., 1981) failed to find significant changes in cortisol as a function of menstrual cycle phase when plasma levels of cortisol were measured on a daily basis. Furthermore, Cudworth and Veevers (1975) and Goldman and Eckerling (1970) assessed glucose tolerance throughout the menstrual cycle and found no variations in glucose tolerance that could be attributed to cycle phase. Although the research concerned with variations in carbohydrate metabolism during the normal menstrual cycle is sparse and several studies were unsuccessful in finding significant variation attributable to the menstrual cycle, the results of those studies that did find significant changes in parameters associated with carbohydrate metabolism are consistent with blood sugar levels being lower during the luteal phase than during the follicular phase.

Since those theorists who attribute some PMS symptoms to hypoglycemia have assumed the source of the hypoglycemia to be abnormal levels of estrogen and/or progesterone (e.g., Dalton, 1964), it would be informative to examine the body of research concerned with the effects of the exogenous administration of hormones, in the form of oral contraceptives and hormone replacement therapy, on carbohydrate metabolism.

Oral contraceptives have been found to cause a reduction in glucose tolerance according to the reports of several investigations (Phillips & Duffy, 1973; Posner, Silverstone, & Tobin, 1975; Goldman & Eckerling, 1970). In contrast, Spellacy and colleagues have found: (a) no consistent changes in blood glucose or plasma insulin in women taking megestrol acetate, an estrogen (Spellacy et al., 1975); (b) normal blood glucose but significantly elevated plasma insulin values in response to norethindrone, a progesterone (Spellacy, Buhi, & Birk, 1975); and (c) significantly lowered fasting glucose values but no change in plasma insulin in women receiving Brevicon—ethinyl estradiol and norethindrone (Spellacy et al., 1982). In these articles, the authors point to progesterone, rather than estrogen, as the source of the changes in carbohydrate metabolism. Spellacy and colleagues (1982) speculated that the type of progestational compound used determines the type and extent of the changes experienced by women ingesting oral contraceptives, but this hypothesis is currently without empirical validation since their studies were not specifically designed to test this hypothesis.

According to the results of two investigations (Amin et al., 1980; Carr et al., 1979), oral contraceptives caused a significant increase in plasma cortisol levels. The latter study found this to be true with drugs containing 50 μg of estrogen, but not 20 μg, implying a dose–response relationship and strongly suggesting that the hormone responsible for the changes in cortisol is estrogen rather than progesterone. Beck and coworkers (1972) and Fern, Rose, and Fern (1978) have reported that the elevation in total plasma cortisol found with oral contraceptives was associated with an estrogen-induced increase in corticosteroid-binding globulin (CBG) concentration. An increase in CBG would cause a greater percentage of the cortisol to be bound and, therefore, be biologically ineffective in providing negative feedback to the hypothalamus and anterior pituitary; as a result of the decreased inhibition, an increase in CRF, ACTH, and, ultimately, cortisol would ensue.

The effects of sex hormones on carbohydrate metabolism have also been studied in the context of hormone replacement therapy for postmenopausal women. Thom and colleagues (1977) found significant deterioration in glucose tolerance, and the degree of deterioration varied according to the content of the medication; patients receiving estradiol valerate and conjugated equine estrogen exhibited the fewest abnormalities. These authors found no change in carbohydrate metabolism as a function of the presence of or the quantity of progesterone. Studd and coworkers (1978) evaluated the effects of a variety of hormone medications given for menopausal symptoms on carbohydrate metabolism. They reported significantly elevated blood glucose for patients receiving estrogen compounds and estrogen plus progesterone compounds, but not for patients receiving progesterone alone. These results suggest that estrogen, rather than progesterone, is the hormone responsible for the abnormalities in carbohydrate metabolism; however, the effects of progesterone on other processes, such as those on the endometrium, are dependent upon previous exposure to estrogen, so progesterone may have actions on carbohydrate metabolism but not independently of estrogen.

Ajabor and colleagues (1972) provided postmenopausal patients with either Premarin (estrogen) or Enovid (estrogen plus progesterone). The effects of these drugs were similar, again suggesting that estrogen is the determinant of the resulting changes. There was a significant deterioration in glucose tolerance at three and six months, but no significant change in insulin secretion or growth hormone. The authors noted that the three subjects who exhibited marked deterioration in tolerance at three months did not exhibit compensatory hyperinsulinism, which does occur in premenopausal women taking oral contraceptives. Thom and coworkers (1977) have pointed out that this failure to compensate with increased insulin may be due to the diminished pancreatic beta-cell reserve with aging.

The effects of hormone replacement therapy on the levels of cortisol were studied by Lobo and colleagues (1982). They administered ACTH to postmenopausal women before and after treatment with estrogen and found that ACTH-stimulated cortisol levels increased after treatment with estrogen. Similar to the results reported above with oral contraceptives, Mahajan and coworkers (1978) found that estrogen replacement therapy resulted in a significant increase in the percentage of bound cortisol; they found increases in CBG, decreases in the metabolic clearance rate of cortisol, and increases in cortisol production rate. The research discussed here suggests that exogenous estrogen results in an increase in plasma cortisol levels, primarily in the form of bound, rather than free, cortisol; and that these changes, in turn, cause a reduction in glucose tolerance.

Di Paola, Robin, and Nicholson (1970) tested the effects of both oral contraceptives and hormone replacement therapy on carbohydrate metabolism; progestrogenic substances had no effect whatsoever, but estrogen compounds caused a decrease in glucose tolerance. The authors pointed out that abnormal glucose tolerance was most frequently seen in women with a family history of diabetes, suggesting that a predisposition may be necessary for such effects to occur. Preston (1971) hypothesized that estrogen increases blood glucose levels in some manner, that this requires an increased need for insulin to prevent hyperglycemia, and that women predisposed to diabetes may be those whose systems are unable to produce the increase in insulin necessary to compensate for the estrogenic effects.

This research on the effects of exogenous hormones on carbohydrate metabolism is difficult to summarize, since the drug, the dosage, the subject population, the length of treatment, and the dependent variables varied from study to study. Such data must clearly be interpreted with caution, since exogenous administration of hormones in the form of oral contraceptives and hormone replacement therapy cause levels of and variations in estrogen and progesterone that differ considerably from those found in normally cycling, unmedicated women. However, one could tentatively conclude that exogenous estrogen tends to cause an increase in blood glucose levels and exogenous progesterone tends to have either no effect or to cause a decrease in blood glucose levels. Integrating these data with the hypothesis that some PMS symptoms may be caused by hypoglycemia would lead to the very tentative conclusion that women suffering from hypoglycemia-induced PMS may have a hormonal imbalance in the luteal phase of the menstrual cycle characterized by elevated levels of progesterone, by diminished levels of estrogen, or by an elevated progesterone–estrogen ratio.

Such a conclusion contradicts the popular belief that PMS is caused by insufficient progesterone or a low progesterone–estrogen ratio (Dalton, 1964). Weideger (1976), on the other hand, has suggested a mechanism by which deficits in progesterone could lead to hypoglycemia. Under normal conditions, progesterone levels are maintained by secretions of the corpus luteum. When insufficient amounts of progesterone are produced for normal cyclic functioning, the reproductive system appropriates progesterone from the adrenal cortex, which produces progesterone as a precursor in the synthesis of corticosteroids. According to this theory, if the adrenal cortex secretes progesterone in response to the body's need, fewer corticosteroids are manufactured. Since a primary corticosteroid is cortisol, which acts to increase the production of glucose and to raise or maintain blood sugar levels, decreases in the synthesis of cortisol as a result of a lack of progesterone may lower blood sugar levels.

The evidence that hypoglycemia occurring during the premenstruum is the cause of premenstrual symptoms and the result of hormonal imbalance is minimal and indirect. The research on the effects of exogenous and endogenous hormones on carbohydrate metabolism is contradictory, and there is a surprising lack of information on carbohydrate metabolism in women suffering from PMS. Considering the striking similarity between the symptoms of hypoglycemia and the symptoms common to PMS, however, and considering the ease of treatment for mild hypoglycemia, such as simple dietary changes, this area deserves considerably more research attention than it has received in the past.

PMS and Prostaglandins

Although prostaglandins have been of considerable interest to researchers and clinicians concerned with menstrual problems, that interest has been limited primarily to the use of prostaglandin inhibitors as a treatment for dysmenorrhea. The idea that prostaglandins may play a role in the etiology of PMS symptoms is relatively recent and has received little attention either at theoretical or at empirical levels. The physiological effects of increased levels of prostaglandins are not limited to those related to uterine contractility. Excess prostaglandin production or the administration of prostaglandins causes nausea, diarrhea, flushing, joint pain, headaches, and breast tenderness (Budoff, 1980; Halbert et al., 1975); each of these prostaglandin-induced effects has been cited as a symptom of PMS.

Because of the similarity between the effects of prostaglandin administration and the symptoms of PMS, drugs that inhibit the synthesis and release of prostaglandins have been tested for their effectiveness in relieving the symptoms of PMS. Wood and Jakubowicz (1980) tested the effectiveness of mefenamic acid in a double-blind crossover design utilizing 39 women suffering from PMS. Each patient completed a symptom checklist daily for three cycles; no medications were administered during the first cycle, and during the second and third cycles patients were given either mefenamic acid or a placebo begun at the first sign of a premenstrual symptom. Of the 37 who completed the study, 23 preferred mefenamic acid over the placebo, and 6 preferred the placebo (8 had no preference). Mefenamic acid was significantly better than placebo at reducing symptoms; the acid effected improvement in tension, irritability, depression, pain, anger, and headaches but did not cause an improvement in breast symptoms and fluid retention.

A similar treatment study has been reported by Budoff (1980). She instructed 43 women suffering from PMS to begin their medications at the onset of their PMS symptoms; for four months, half took Ponstel, a prostaglandin inhibitor, and half a placebo; they then crossed over and took the other medication. During the cycles in which the women took the prostaglandin inhibitor, they reported significantly less breast tenderness, abdominal bloating, menstrual pain, and nausea when compared to placebo cycles; there was no improvement in tension, lethargy, or depression.

Although there is no direct evidence linking prostaglandins to PMS symptomatology, the two treatment studies are promising, and such treatment is logically consistent with the fact that endometrial prostaglandins exhibit a dramatic increase during the late luteal phase at about the time when PMS symptoms appear (Singh et al., 1975; Willman et al., 1976). There is also evidence to suggest that progesterone tends to inhibit prostaglandin synthesis (Cane & Villee, 1975). Thus, the prostaglandin theory of PMS may be viewed as being consistent with the popular view that PMS is due to a lack of progesterone, since a lack of progesterone may result in excess prostaglandins, and treatment with either progesterone or prostaglandin inhibitors may cause a decrease in symptoms via a decrease in prostaglandins.

PMS and Endogenous Opiates

A new and highly promising theory on the biochemical etiology of PMS involves endogenous opiates. Endogenous opiates are neuropeptides that exhibit pharmacological properties similar to morphine. Two such substances—enkephalins and endorphins—have been isolated; of these, beta-endorphin is the major and most potent naturally stored product. These neuropeptides are elaborated by the pituitary and act on the central and peripheral nervous systems to reduce pain.

Evidence suggests that endorphin concentrations vary with the menstrual cycle. Reid and Yen (1981) cite one study that demonstrated endorphin levels to be high during the midluteal phase and undetectable at the beginning of menses in rhesus monkeys. Evidence for variations associated with the menstrual cycle in humans is indirect. Endorphin levels appear to play a role in the release of gonadotropins, probably by inhibiting hypothalamic GnRH activity. Reid, Hoff, and Yen (1981) noted a significant decrease in LH concentrations in both men and women after administering synthetic endorphin. Quigley and Yen (1980) administered the opiate antagonist, naloxone, and observed a significant increase in LH release in both the late follicular and midluteal phases of the cycle; there was no obvious effect of LH concentrations during the early follicular phase. Data consistent with these were reported by Robert, Quigley, and Yen (1981), who infused naloxone during the luteal phase; the subjects exhibited an increase both in frequency and in amplitude of LH pulses and a significant increment in FSH levels. One interpretation of such findings is that, since endorphins affect LH levels and since the inhibition of endorphins with naloxone appears to influence LH levels only during the late follicular and luteal phases, then it seems probable that endorphin concentrations are higher during the luteal phase than during the follicular phase.

Fritz and Speroff (1983) cite evidence indicating that the cyclic fluctuations in endogenous opiates are the result of endogenous levels of estrogen and progesterone. Exogenous estrogen administered to ovariectomized monkeys had no consistent effect on portal endorphin levels; but the administration of both estrogen and progesterone, the hormone pattern typical of the luteal phase, induced large increases in levels of endorphins in the portal blood. They concluded that ". . . the observation that portal endorphin concentrations are highest in the luteal phase and can be elevated by the combined administration of estradiol and progesterone implicates the action of endogenous opiates in the reduced pulse frequency of gonadotropin secretion during the luteal phase" (p. 675). Thus, endorphin levels appear to vary systematically with the menstrual cycle, concentrations of estrogen and progesterone may modify endorphin production and release, and one action of endorphins may be to influence the level and pulse amplitude of LH.

These data, along with the well-known effects of exogenous opiates and withdrawal from the chronic use of opiates, led Reid and Yen (1981, 1983) to develop a theoretical model of PMS in which the causal agent is the changing level of endogenous opiates during the menstrual cycle: "We postulate that an aberrant release of, or sensitivity to, the neurointermediate lobe peptides a-MSH and B-endorphin during the luteal phase may be the central event which triggers a cascade of neuroendocrine changes leading ultimately to the varied manifestations of the PMS" (Reid & Yen, 1983, p. 713).

Of potential importance in tying PMS to levels of endogenous opiates is the research on the relationship between endorphins and stress. To summarize a discussion in an earlier chapter, endogenous opiates are the crucial biochemicals involved in a phenomenon referred to as stress-induced analgesia (SIA). SIA involves a decrease in pain sensitivity following exposure to stimuli that are psychologically stressful. One form of SIA is mediated by endogenous opiates, and this is the form that is induced when the organism is exposed to chronic, uncontrollable stressors. Furthermore, SIA may be classically conditioned so that endogenous opiates may be released prior to the stressor if the stressor is predictable.

To extend, in a purely speculative fashion, the theory proposed by Reid and Yen (1983), menstruation may be viewed as a chronic and uncontrollable, but predictable, event that is stressful for some women either because they experience painful menstruation, because they subscribe to the cultural taboos surrounding menstruation, and/or because they feel it necessary to abstain from enjoyable experiences such as exercise or sex. For those women who view menstruation as stressful, the levels of endogenous opiates during the premenstruum, which are normally elevated at this time, may reach even higher levels as a result of the conditioned release of endorphins in response to the impending menstrual period. The abnormally high levels of endogenous opiates may be accompanied by symptoms typical of this physiological state, such as increased appetite. In addition, endogenous opiates may trigger a variety of neuroendocrine events, leading ultimately to the symptoms commonly associated with PMS. For example, endogenous opiates tend to inhibit the production of neurotransmitters in the central nervous system (Reid & Yen, 1981), and reductions of these neurotransmitters are typically associated with fatigue and depression. Furthermore, endorphin-induced inhibition of the neurotransmitter, dopamine, may cause an increased release of prolactin (Reid et al., 1981), which would increase fluid retention and, possibly, cause weight gain and breast tenderness. Furthermore, the subsequent decline in endorphins caused by the rapidly falling levels of estrogen and progesterone during the premenstruum may result in symptoms similar to those associated with withdrawal from morphine, such as irritability, anxiety, tension, and aggression.

Furthermore, the conditioned release of endorphins prior to menstruation may increase in strength over the years, resulting in less painful menstruation due to the opiate-induced analgesia and more severe PMS symptoms; this would be consistent with research findings that PMS increases and dysmenorrhea decreases with age. Finally, endorphin release has been suggested as the mediating mechanism responsible for the effectiveness of placebos in reducing pain (Watkins & Mayer, 1982)—that is, if one expects a placebo to reduce pain, this may evoke a conditioned endorphin response, which would, in fact, cause pain reduction. Such a phenomenon could explain the frequently significant improvement in PMS symptoms in response to placebos.

The relationship between endogenous opiates and PMS will undoubtedly generate considerable research interest. If their theory receives empirical validation, Reid and Yen (1981) suggest new possibilities for treatment, such as the narcotic antagonist, naltrexone, or the a-adrenergic agonist, clonidine; both may be useful in counteracting the manifestations of opiate withdrawal. Interestingly, progesterone, which as a treatment for PMS has generated considerable controversy during the last 20 years, may prove to be a logical treatment choice, since it, in conjunction with estrogen, has been shown in preliminary studies to increase levels of endogenous endorphins.

Summary

The most popular physiological theory of PMS hypothesizes reduced progesterone or high estrogen–progesterone ratio to be etiological. Studies that have found progesterone to be lower in women with PMS than in those who are symptom-free, or those that have found estrogen levels to be positively correlated with symptoms, offer support for this theory. Furthermore, the theory is a logical one for some symptoms in that low levels of progesterone can cause changes such as elevations in prolactin and decreased blood sugar; however, there is little evidence that these mechanisms actually do operate to cause premenstrual symptoms. Finally, the treatment effectiveness of progesterone for PMS is not impressive, particularly when compared to the effectiveness of other treatments, such as diuretics or even placebos.

Research and clinical reports concerned with the physiological etiology of PMS have yielded contradictory results and left many questions unanswered. Inconsistent and contradictory results are, perhaps, to be expected, given the idiosyncratic procedures for assessing biochemical, endocrinological, and psychological variables and given the variety of populations sampled. On the other hand, the confusion apparent in the published literature could well be a reflection of the enormous complexity of the problem.

One criticism of this body of research is the narrow focus of most investigations. Interactions among systems hypothesized to be etiologically related to PMS are generally ignored. Several examples will serve to illustrate. Both MAO levels and hypoglycemia have been implicated in the development of premenstrual depression, but MAO inhibitors have been shown to induce hypoglycemia; norepinephrine, which is assumed to vary inversely with MAO, tends to inhibit insulin release; and aldosterone affects both fluid retention and carbohydrate metabolism (Hall et al., 1974). Thus, restricting one's attention to the association between premenstrual symptoms and one's favorite dependent variable is likely to provide an incomplete view of the actual relationships.

Related to this issue are potential interactions between environmental stress and hypothesized physiological mechanisms. Psychological trauma or stress can elevate serum prolactin levels (Mason, 1975), increase the formation of glucocorticoids, which, in turn, effect changes in blood sugar level (Navratil, 1975), deplete norepinephrine (Miller & Weiss, 1969), increase MAO levels (Weiss et al., 1979), cause elevated levels of endorphins (Akil et al., 1984), and lower gonadotropin production to the point of inducing amenorrhea (Check, 1978). In none of the studies discussed above was stress or the effect of stress on the relationship between physiological factors and PMS symptoms assessed.

The strong possibility exists that PMS is a heterogeneous disorder both in terms of etiology and symptomatology. The only reason for combining symptoms such as depression, irritability, sluggishness, restlessness, and swelling under the title of PMS is because of the assumed temporal relationship to the menstrual cycle. To my knowledge, no research has addressed the questions of how many symptoms have to be experienced premenstrually to warrant a diagnosis of PMS, whether some combinations of symptoms appear with a greater frequency than others, or whether the same symptoms are experienced during each premenstrual phase in the same woman. Indeed, it is possible and likely that the various symptoms have different causes. There is no reason to expect that depression and water retention share a common etiology, nor should it be assumed that both will respond to the same treatment. Improved methods of assessing symptomatology, along with the recognition that PMS may consist of several distinct syndromes, are indicated for future research.

9

The Current Popularity
of PMS

A discussion of PMS would be incomplete without attention to the recent intense interest in PMS among professional and lay persons. PMS was the disease of the year in 1982, as evidenced by the coverage it received in popular paperbacks, talk shows, and magazines. The reasons for this interest are not readily apparent. Perhaps it was due to two highly publicized murder cases in which British women received reduced sentences because it was considered that PMS rendered them incapacitated and irresponsible; or it could be that Katherine Dalton's (1964) view of PMS as a hormonal disorder treatable by progesterone caught on in the United States. Irrespective of the reasons, the consequence of this popularity has been a change toward viewing PMS as a legitimate medical disorder.

One topic of current interest concerns PMS as a precipitator of violent crime. An early study by Dalton (1961) is frequently cited as evidence for an increase in criminal activity during the premenstrual phase. In a group of women prisoners, significantly more of their crimes had occurred during the paramenstruum (premenstrual plus menstrual phases) than during the rest of the cycle. Statistics were not reported separately for the menstrual and the premenstrual phases, so it is unclear whether these data support a premenstrual increase in crime. Furthermore, 44% of the paramenstrual crimes were ones of prostitution; and the temporal relationship of this crime to the menstrual cycle may have been due to the relative risk of pregnancy. In a more recent study, d'Orban and Dalton (1980) interviewed 50 women prisoners; significantly more women than expected by chance had committed their crimes during the paramenstruum, but when the data were analyzed separately for premenstrual and menstrual phases, only the menstrual phase frequencies were significantly higher than those in the remaining days of the cycle. Of the 17 women who complained of PMS, 29% had committed their crimes during the paramenstruum, which is about what one would expect by chance. In both of these studies, as in the studies of suicide and the menstrual cycle discussed in an earlier chapter, women who could not remember the time of their menses were eliminated from subject samples—a procedure that could bias the sample in the direction of including those women who were menstruating at the time of the crime.

On the other hand, Dalton (1980) has extensively documented three cases in which women suffering from PMS had acted in an irrational, bizarre, and criminal manner, and such behaviors occurred consistently during the premenstrual phase and not during other phases of the cycle. In all three cases, high doses of progesterone improved or eliminated the cyclic behavior. Thus, although one can find instances of criminal behavior that are apparently related to the menstrual cycle, there is no empirical support for the idea that women, in general, are more likely to commit crimes during the premenstrual phase, or even that women who commit crimes are more likely to do so during this phase. As in other areas of menstrual cycle research, conclusions regarding the relationship between the menstrual cycle and crime have been magnified beyond the actual empirical data.

As a direct consequence of Dalton's work, the use of PMS as a legal defense has been argued successfully in England, and two women have received reduced sentences contingent upon their continuing treatment for PMS. If one accepts temporary or permanent mental disability as an appropriate defense, then there is no reason, theoretically, for not including mental instability due to PMS as a defense. However, the diagnoses of PMS in the two British women are not consistent with current scientific views. For example, in order for these women to be considered PMS sufferers, it had to be demonstrated that their premenstrual violent behaviors were eliminated with progesterone treatment, and, clearly, not all women who suffer from PMS are successfully treated with progesterone.

Of considerable concern to feminists are the consequences of excusing violent behavior when it is viewed as a symptom of PMS. The potential for increased discrimination against women was ex-

pressed by Sommer (1984): "If PMS is a function of women's reproductive physiology, then theoretically any menstruating woman has
an excuse for irrational behavior" (p. 37), and "If the courts, working
hand-in-hand with science, appear to confirm this long-held view of
women as hapless victims of their biological nature, neither the
legal system nor the medical system nor society at large will be well
served" (p. 38). Although the concern is a legitimate one, the threat
of generalizing from a few women criminals who plead PMS as a
defense to women in general is only possible because such generali-
zations are consistent with the negative stereotypes of women as
intellectually inferior and biologically determined.

One consequence of the new popularity of PMS has been the
establishment of specialized clinics to treat PMS. Unfortunately, the
proliferation of these clinics has not been associated with the development of improved treatment methods. According to a gynecolo-
gist employed by one of the PMS clinics, all clients are advised ". . .
to cut down on salt and sugar to reduce water retention, and he
sometimes prescribes vitamin B6 and exercise. If anxiety and nervousness persist, he goes to progesterone therapy . . ." (Heneson,
1984, p. 68). All of these methods of treatment for PMS have been
recognized for the last 20 years, and all are somewhat effective, as
discussed above; none, however, produce miracle cures. On the
positive side, many women afflicted with PMS had previously suffered in silence and were unaware of even the simplest modes of
treatment such as dietary changes. The new-found popularity of
PMS has resulted in women feeling more comfortable in seeking
medical treatment without the fear that they would be dismissed as
neurotic, and, although the treatments recommended are not new,
their widespread use is.

The 1982 explosion of interest in PMS is already dying down.
Many of the PMS clinics have closed, and the popular literature on
the subject has become skeptical. A recent article in *Psychology
Today* (Hopson & Rosenfeld, 1984) states that progesterone treatment for PMS was accepted too readily, has potentially negative
side effects, and has not been proven to be superior to placebos. At
approximately the same time, an article appeared in the magazine
Science 84 (Heneson, 1984), which presented a rather cynical view
of PMS clinics and described them as a way for unreputable persons
to become rich by offering treatment of questionable value to unsus-
pecting women. In support of her skeptical view of these clinics,
Heneson reported that a physician employed at a PMS clinic stated
that a lack of sufficient progesterone results in the body accumula-

ting fluid, and the fluid retention causes anxiety; the evidence he gave to support this contention was that there are more murders on hot, humid days.

Although the popular interest in PMS and the proliferation of commercial PMS clinics seems to be diminishing, the acceptance of PMS by the medical community has spurred new research endeavors among gynecologists, neurologists, endocrinologists, and psychologists in the search for causes and treatments. Research currently in progress is indicative of the increasing awareness of the deficiencies of past research in that important issues are being addressed, such as the validity of retrospective self-reports, interactions among the potentially relevant physiological systems, the impact of environmental stress, and the importance of placebo comparisons in assessing treatment effectiveness.

10

Future Directions

The research findings discussed in this chapter are theoretically consistent with an organic etiology of PMS and dysmenorrhea. Fluctuations in estrogen and progesterone associated with the normal menstrual cycle can and do affect the synthesis and release of substances in the central nervous system, the pituitary, and the reproductive tract, which, in turn, have a potential impact on water retention, mood, carbohydrate metabolism, vasomotor activity, arousal, and myometrial activity. Given the tremendous complexity of these interdependent physiological systems, the potential for dysfunction is great. Minor changes in sensitivity to a particular hormone or modifications in the synthesis and release of a particular substance could be manifest in a multitude of symptoms ranging from abdominal pain to severe depression, and they could be due to a variety of causes ranging from an inadequate diet to a metabolic disorder.

The lack of support for a psychological etiology of PMS and dysmenorrhea is perhaps due to a limited perspective constricted by traditional and stereotypic views of women in our society. Until very recently, researchers and theoreticians interested in a psychological perspective of menstrual disorders have concentrated on general neurotic traits and/or a lack of femininity—neither of which seems to bear a significant relationship to menstrual disorders. However, defining psychological causes as transitory states brought about or exacerbated by stress opens entirely new vistas for research on the etiology of menstrual disorders. Although empirical work relating stress and menstrual disorders is lacking, there is considerable evidence suggestive of the potential for stress to influence significantly factors associated with menstrual distress. For example, since the uterine muscle and vessels supplying the blood to the uterine muscle are innvervated by the autonomic nervous system, sympathetic arousal or increased levels of plasma catecholamines brought about by stress could result in increased contractility of the muscle and/or vasoconstriction of the blood vessels. Similarly, stress has been shown to be associated with increased levels of endorphins, monoamine oxidase, prolactin, and cortisol—all of which have been linked to at least one symptom of PMS.

Of obvious relevance to a theory that hypothesizes stress as etiological in menstrual disorders is the issue of temporal contiguity—why would stress be more likely to occur during the paramenstruum than at other times during the cycle, or why does stress not produce similar symptoms during other phases of the cycle? Only speculative answers to these questions are currently possible, but, since stress undoubtedly occurs throughout the menstrual cycle, it is possible that the particular biochemical profile characteristic of the premenstrual or menstrual phases renders one particularly vulnerable to stress and/or to developing particular symptoms—those typical of PMS or dysmenorrhea. On the other hand, subjective stress may well increase during the paramenstruum as a result of the sociocultural views of menstruation—that it is dirty, a form of illness, debilitating, and an embarrassment—having been internalized.

Thus, the research investigating the etiology of menstrual disorders is theoretically consistent with either an organic or a stress etiology; empirical evidence in both areas is limited in that the potential for causation has been demonstrated but evidence conclusively linking either or both to menstrual disorders is lacking. Furthermore, advocating one etiological mechanism to the exclusion of others is not as potentially productive as theories allowing for the mutually interactive and additive effects of various causes. A model previously proposed by Akiskal (1979) to account for the effects of various factors in the etiology of depression may be useful in conceptualizing menstrual disorders. Akiskal proposed an optimally functioning diencephalic reward system as the final common pathway in the etiology of depression; that is, any event—whether psychological, environmental, or physiological—that reduces opti-mal functioning in this center increases the vulnerability to depres-sion.

Applying such a model to menstrual disorders requires speci-fying a final common pathway and then determining which factors impact on that pathway. For example, the final common pathway for dysmenorrheic cramps may be elevated levels of prostaglandins; any event or process that results in elevated prostaglandin levels increases one's vulnerability to menstrual cramps. The possible direct causes of elevated levels of prostaglandins include elevated levels of estrogen, insufficient progesterone, cervical obstruction, large fragments of endometrium in the menstrual product, increased levels of oxytocin and/or vasopressin, and increased muscle tension due to stress and mediated by the autonomic nervous system. These factors may be secondarily influenced by a variety of factors inclu-ding genetically transmitted abnormalities, inadequate diet, syste-mic disease, and trauma. Finally, interactive and additive effects among these variables may influence the probability of developing menstrual disorders. The appeal of this model is that it diverts the focus away from an unproductive search for the one cause, implies logical targets for treatment interventions, and acknowledges the potential for multiple causation both within and across individuals.

The treatment research presents an even more imposing task in terms of integration. All of the present medical treatments for both dysmenorrhea and PMS are symptomatic—that is, the goal is to relieve symptoms rather than to alter underlying abnormalities—and since causes are not altered, medication must be taken on a continuous basis. Moreover, studies that evaluate the effectiveness of such treatments do not contribute, on a theoretical level, to the understanding of etiology. Psychological treatment generally at-tempts to cure, but there is simply too little of this research to allow adequate evaluation. A further issue relates to the treatment of PMS. Studies have typically found a particular treatment to be effective for some women and not for others. For example, diuretics may be found to alleviate symptoms for only a third of a particular sample and are, therefore, dismissed as ineffective. However, while diure-tics may not be effective for those women whose primary symptom is depression, they may be so for those whose primary symptom is water retention. For future research, logic dictates the use of samples that are homogeneous in symptomatology. This view concurs with that of previous authors, who have concluded that

PMS is most likely to consist of several disorders with distinct etiologies, symptoms, and preferred treatments.

As with most disorders considered to have both organic and stress-related etiologies, research on menstrual disorders is directed by a variety of individuals who represent a diversity of levels and types of training. Most of the literature on menstrual disorders may be classified into two general categories: One type of research, which tends to be most common in studies employing psychological variables, involves the use of appropriate control groups in standard experimental designs and employs sophisticated statistical analyses but fails to employ adequate methods for determining cycle phase or hormonal levels. The other type of research, typical of studies employing physiological variables, may be commended for careful hormonal analyses and valid methods for determining time of ovulation, but is clearly lacking in appropriate experimental design and statistical analyses; frequently, phenomena are observed and reported, with no indication as to the likelihood of these observations occurring by chance.

A solution would be to relax the barriers separating the various disciplines and to encourage collaboration among researchers with various specializations. Hopefully, this would not only generate studies free from the above criticisms but facilitate an appreciation for the interactions among environmental, sociocultural, psychological, and physiological causes and a willingness to accept that the understanding and treatment of menstrual disorders requires complex, rather than simple, solutions.

THE MENOPAUSAL SYNDROME

Introduction

"Menopause," strictly speaking, refers to the cessation of menstruation. The term "climacteric" refers to the transition period between middle and old age and applies to physical and emotional changes that occur both in women and in men during this time period. Although "climacteric syndrome" would be a more accurate term for the symptoms associated with the years preceding and subsequent to menopause, "menopausal syndrome" is the term popularly used. Ovarian failure, which ultimately culminates in menopause, is a gradual process lasting five to ten years. It is believed that by the time a woman reaches her early forties, the number of remaining follicles is considerably reduced, and that those remaining exhibit a lessened responsiveness to gonadotropin stimulation (Studd, Chakravarti, & Oram, 1977). As a result, during some menstrual cycles, follicular development may not occur, which, in turn, results in somewhat lowered levels of estrogen, elevated levels of follicle-stimulating hormone (FSH) and luteinizing hormone (LH), a lack of ovulation, and an irregular pattern of bleeding. Typically, as this transitional period progesses, more and more cycles are anovulatory, until menses stops completely. Symptoms commonly associated with the menopausal syndrome may begin at any time during this transitional period.

Much of the research on the menopausal syndrome has been designed and interpreted within a theoretical framework in which the menopause itself is viewed as a disease. Such an orientation has been pervasive in both the popular and scientific literature and is evidenced by statements such as "It has been suggested, with an admitted lack of reverence, that the menopause is a biologic accident and that women were perhaps not originally destined to live for as many years postmenopausally as modern medical science now permits" (Rogers, 1956, p. 699). Not only has medical science advanced somewhat since 1956, but so have our perspectives on women and women's roles. However, despite scientific advances and social enlightenment, menopause continues to be viewed as an unnatural and pathological condition characterized by a variety of negative physical and psychological symptoms believed to be due to a deficiency of estrogen.

It seems inappropriate to consider a process that occurs in every woman as anything but natural. By suggesting that menopause is a natural event, I do not mean to imply that physiological changes do not occur, nor that some of these changes are not accompanied by distress and discomfort. However, other events in women's lives, such as pregnancy and menarche, are associated with physiological changes and are frequently accompanied by pain and psychological distress; but these events are not viewed as disorders nor as undesirable physiological processes, but as natural events that occasionally require treatment for associated symptoms. As Posner (1979) noted, it is ironical that, if menstruation is considered a curse, as the professional and popular literature suggest, then menopause is not considered a blessing.

In the following chapters, two menopausal symptoms have been singled out for extensive discussion—hot flashes and osteoporosis. Hot flashes were selected for special consideration because they are the most common menopausal complaint and the most common symptom treated. In addition, there has been a dramatic increase in the last decade in research into the causes of hot flashes. Osteoporosis, a condition characterized by the loss of bone density and an increased susceptibility to fractures, was selected because it is considered to be a menopausal symptom, and the prevention of osteoporosis is frequently the rationale given for treating all women with hormones from the time of menopause until the end of their lives.

11

The Endocrinology of Menopause

The hormonal changes that occur during menopause probably originate with a lessened ability of the ovary to produce estrogen and progesterone, and the cause of this decrease in hormonal production is assumed to be due to a reduction in the follicles available for stimulation (Studd, Chakravarti, & Oram, 1977). The decreased levels of estrogen result in a loss of negative feedback to the hypothalamus and, in turn, to the pituitary; the loss of this negative feedback is assumed to be the cause of the elevated levels of LH and FSH typical of the menopausal and postmenopausal years (Smith, Rodriquez-Rigdu, & Steinberger, 1981).

The menopausal process is not a sudden one in natural menopause but a gradual decrease in ovulatory cycles, with increasing levels of LH and FSH and decreasing levels of estrogen until menstruation ceases completely; this usually occurs between the ages of 45 and 55. Adamopoulos, Loraine, and Dove (1971) studied a group of premenopausal women, aged 37 to 42; these women had LH levels approximately seven times greater and FSH levels approximately three times greater than those found in younger women, along with reduced levels of estrogen and progesterone. The authors expressed surprise at the existence of such high levels of gonadotropins in the absence of menopausal symptoms and in the presence of ovulation. In a similar study, Sherman, West, and Korenman (1976) found lowered estradiol concentrations, increased FSH concentrations, but LH concentrations in the normal range in a group of women approaching menopause. Such data argue against the theory that gonadotropins increase as a result of ovarian failure; however, Hammond and Dry (1982) speculate that perhaps, given the reduced number of follicles, an increased level of FSH is required to promote follicular development.

In contrast to this typically gradual process, surgical removal of the ovaries in premenopausal women produces an abrupt menopause. Shortly after surgery, estrogen levels fall dramatically, and gonadotropin levels gradually increase (Hunter et al., 1977; Ostergard, Parlow, & Townsend, 1970; Utian et al., 1978). Monroe, Jaffe, and Midgley (1972) reported that in their sample FSH levels initially rose more rapidly than LH levels and that, at one month following surgery, the elevated gonadotropin levels had not yet reached postmenopausal levels in all subjects.

Estrogen Production during the Climacteric Transition

The postmenopausal ovary is not totally inactive in terms of hormone production. The ovary is divided into two areas: the outer cortex contains granulosa cells that are the primary source of ovarian estrogen (Longcope, Hunter, & Franz, 1980); these cells are decreased in number and productive capacity after menopause. However, the ovarian stroma, which is capable of synthesizing the androgens—androstenedione, dehydroepiandrosterone, and testosterone—continues hormone production after menopause, and these compounds may undergo peripheral conversion to estrogen (Hunter, 1976). Several lines of evidence suggest that the postmenopausal ovary secretes little if any estrogen. Mattingly and Huang (1969) assessed the steroidogenesis of ovarian tissue slices taken from menopausal and postmenopausal women. This tissue was clearly capable of producing dehydroepiandrosterone and testosterone, but it yielded minimal amounts of estrone and estradiol. Furthermore, the similarity between estrogen levels of women with natural versus surgical menopause implies that estrogen is not being secreted by the ovaries (Radar et al., 1973).

More direct data regarding the hormone production of the postmenopausal ovary comes from a study by Judd and colleagues (1974). They compared the concentrations of testosterone, androstenedione, estradiol, and estrone in peripheral and ovarian vein blood taken from ten postmenopausal women. A higher concentration of all these hormones was found in the ovarian vein than in the peripheral vein; the magnitude of the differences were 15-fold for testosterone, 4-fold for androstenedione, and 2-fold for both estradiol and estrone. The authors concluded that the postmenopausal ovary secretes primarily androgens while retaining a minimal amount of estrogen secretion. Mattingly and Huang (1969) have suggested that this continued androgen production may contribute to the minor androgenic state of postmenopausal women, including balding on the scalp, hair growth on the face and chest, and subcutaneous fat distribution.

Despite the evidence that the ovaries cease to secrete other than possibly minimal amounts of estrogen after menopause, estrogen can be detected in the plasma of postmenopausal women. The mechanism of estrogen production in postmenopausal women is believed to be the aromatization of androstenedione in peripheral tissue, particularly adipose tissue. Data consistent with this hypothesis have been reported in several studies (Judd, Lucas, & Yen, 1976; Rader et al., 1973; Vermeulen, 1976), which found estradiol and estrone levels not to be significantly different in oophorectomized women and postmenopausal women with ovaries. Hunter (1976) suggested that although the ovarian stroma is capable of synthesizing androstenedione, these cells do not secrete estrogen, and although removal of the ovaries results in a 50% reduction in circulating androstenedione, there is not a corresponding change in estrone because the rate of peripheral conversion is increased to make up for the difference.

Research investigating the percentage of total estrogen that is the product of peripheral conversion has not yielded consistent results. In one study (Grodin, Siiteri, & MacDonald, 1973), the quantity of estrone derived from aromatization of androgens was essentially the same as the absolute levels of estrone, suggesting that all estrone was derived in this manner. In contrast, Judd and coworkers (1982) assessed the metabolic clearance rate, conversion ratios, and production rates of androgens, estrone, and estradiol. The peripheral conversion of androgens accounted for 24.6% of circulating estrone but only for minimal quantities of estradiol, while the peripheral conversion of estrone accounted for 21.5% of estradiol. The subjects in this study had intact ovaries, but the research cited above suggests that it is unlikely that the ovaries are the source of the estogens unaccounted for by peripheral conversion. Age may be a factor of relevance to this issue. Hemsell and coworkers (1974) found significant relationships between the efficiency of conversion and age, indicating that, as one ages, the body becomes more efficient at converting androgens to estrogens. It is interesting that

significant correlations between conversion rate and age were reported for both men and women, although the correlation for women
was higher.

The research discussed above indicates that the postmenopausal woman has detectable levels of estrogen in her plasma, that the
presence or absence of ovaries does not seem to influence significantly the levels of circulating estrogens, and that the peripheral
conversion of androgens to estrogen, although a major source of
estrogen, may not account for all estrogen. Since the adrenal cortex
is capable of synthesizing and secreting androgens, this gland may
also be capable of synthesizing estrogen or may contribute significantly to the pool of precursors available for peripheral conversion.
Several studies have reported a minimal change in circulating levels
of estrone after oophorectomy, although androgens were found to
decrease (Chang & Judd, 1981; Vermeulen, 1976). Such data suggest
that the adrenal cortex may secrete estrogens. Some researchers
have stimulated the adrenal cortex with adrenocorticotrophic hormone (ACTH) and found significant increases in estrone, progesterone, and androstenedione (Murakami, Yamaji, & Ohsawa, 1976;
Poliak et al., 1971; Vermeulen, 1976). Both Murakami and colleagues and Maroulis and Abraham (1976) interpreted such data to
mean that the adrenal cortex directly secretes estrone, although this
is difficult to determine conclusively since increases in estrone may
be due to increased peripheral conversion of androgens to estrone.
To summarize, the adrenal cortex seems to be a major source of
estrone in the postmenopausal women, but it is not clear whether
estrone is secreted directly or whether the adrenals secrete androgens, which are then converted to estrogen.

Adipose tissue is a primary site of the peripheral conversion of
testosterone and androstenedione to estradiol and estrone in postmenopausal women (Archer, 1982). This process is believed to be
the underlying cause of the consistent finding that circulating levels
of estrone and estradiol are significantly correlated with body
weight and excess fat in postmenopausal women (Badawy et al.,
1979; Judd, Lucas, & Yen, 1976). Although levels of estrogen would
be, in theory, due to the availability of precursors and the rate of
conversion, weight has not been found to correlate with circulating
androstenedione and testosterone levels, so the association between
weight and estrogen levels is assumed to be due to the increased rate
of conversion, which, in turn, is possible because of the greater
amount of fat.

Weight has also been found to be negatively correlated with the
circulating concentration of sex-hormone-binding globulin (SHBG),

a plasma protein that binds with estradiol and renders it biologically inactive (Erlik, Meldrum, & Judd, 1982). Thus, body fat appears to have a dual effect on estrogen levels: excess body fat is associated with an increased conversion of androgens to estrogens, and the lower levels of SHBG exhibited by obese persons suggest that less estrogen is bound, and more is active, than in thin persons. These processes are presumed to account for the greater incidence of hot flashes and osteoporosis among thin postmenopausal women than among the obese.

Gonadotropin Production during the Climacteric Transition

There is confusion in the literature as to the cause of the elevated levels of gonadotropins after menopause. Given the feedback mechanisms necessary for normal menstrual cycling during the premenopausal years, it is possible that: (a) the decreasing levels of estrogen cause diminished negative feedback to the hypothalamus, resulting in greater production of gonadotropin-releasing hormone (GnRH); (b) the levels of GnRH remain the same, but the sensitivity of the pituitary to GnRH increases, resulting in greater production of LH and FSH; or (c) both hypothalamic and pituitary activity is similar to that of premenopausal years, but the metabolic clearance rates of LH and FSH are reduced. Rosenblum and Schlaff (1976) reported levels of GnRH in postmenopausal women to be undetectable and concluded that the elevated levels of gonadotropins in postmenopausal women were the result of an increase in pituitary sensitivity due to low levels of estrogen. However, Archer (1982) has suggested that hypothalamic GnRH is released in a pulsatile manner, and high levels could easily be overlooked unless blood was sampled frequently.

In support of Archer's view, Seyler and Reichlin (1973) sampled blood every ten minutes for several hours and found GnRH in postmenopausal women frequently to be in the range of premenopausal values, but seven of the 25 women exhibited values greater than three standard deviations higher. Similarly, Henrik (1982) cites evidence to indicate an increase in levels of GnRH in the menopausal and postmenopausal years. The variability of values found for GnRH in postmenopausal women may well be due to the episodic nature of the release, which is also apparent in the cyclic, pulsatile discharge of FSH and LH from the pituitary at intervals of 60 to 70

minutes. Similar pulses of FSH and LH are present during menar-
chal years, but the amplitude of the pulses is smaller, and the
periodicity is asynchronous compared to menopausal women (Archer, 1982).

Menopause versus Aging

Since menopause typically occurs in women between the ages of 45
and 55, some of the physiological changes that have been attributed
to the menopause may, in fact, be due to the aging process. If
endocrinological changes are primarily due to aging, then one
would expect to find a significant relationship between the levels of
various hormones and age; if such endocrinological changes are due
to menopause, on the other hand, the relationship between hormone levels and age would be absent, and one would expect to find
relatively constant levels prior to menopause, an abrupt shift coincident with menopause, and relatively constant levels subsequent to
menopause. The patterns noted for estrogen are consistent with a
menopausal hypothesis—that is, estrogen levels decrease at the
time of menopause but are not significantly correlated with age or
years since menopause (Judd, Lucas, & Yen, 1976; Judd et al., 1980;
Meldrum et al., 1981a; Reyes, Winter, & Faiman, 1977).

In contrast, Meldrum and colleagues (1981a) assessed hormonal levels in women aged 34 to 83, all of whom had experienced
menopause but had intact ovaries. They found a strong negative
relationship between levels of the androgens dehydroepiandrosterone (DHEA) and dehydroepiandrosterone sulfate (DHEAS) with
age; androstendedione and testosterone were significantly lower
than levels found in premenopausal women, but levels of these
androgens were uncorrelated with age. These authors concluded
that adrenal androgen secretion decreases as a function of age.
Cumming and coworkers (1982) measured circulating DHEAS in
women with premature ovarian failure, after ovariectomy, and subsequent to menopause. They found that premature ovarian failure
and ovariectomy in young as well as postmenopausal subjects precipitated an earlier decline in DHEAS levels and concluded that the
decline in DHEAS is a function of both age and ovarian failure,
whether it be due to natural or surgical menopause.

Finally, the effects of age versus menopause on levels of FSH
and LH have been investigated. Reyes, Winter, and Faiman (1977)
reported that while FSH exhibited a significant correlation with age,

LH did not but was considerably higher postmenopause than pre-menopause. The obvious explanation for elevated levels of LH and FSH in postmenopausal women is the absence of negative feedback due to lowered levels of estrogen associated with ovarian failure. However, Henrik (1982) suggests there may also be age-related physiological changes which would tend to enhance the increased gonadotropin levels even further. One such change is a decreasing ability of the aging organism to inactivate or excrete LH from the circulation, which would result in accumulation of gonadotropins; another mechanism may be a reduction in the hormone-binding capacity of the brain due to aging, which would decrease the negative feedback effects of the estrogen that is present in the circulation. Thus, the elevated levels of gonadotropins evident in the postmenopausal women may be due primarily to the diminished production of estrogen but may be enhanced by other age-related physiological processes.

In summary, natural menopause is a gradual process, with a progressive increase in anovulatory cycles and eventual cessation of menses. The hormonal changes accompanying this process probably originate with a decrease in estrogen production by the ovaries, and the lowered levels of estrogen act to increase levels of the gonadotropins. Although estrogen is usually detectable in postmenopausal women, the primary source of these estrogens is probably the peripheral conversion of androgen, with minimal amounts of estrogen directly secreted by the ovaries or the adrenal cortex. Although the inactive ovaries of menopausal women are probably the major determinant of the shift in the hormonal profile in elderly women, other factors, such as physiological changes due to aging and percentage of body fat, are contributory.

12

Menopausal Symptoms

Not only is menopause viewed as an indication of aging in a culture where youth is highly valued, but the popularized version of the "menopausal syndrome" consists of a variety of clearly unpleasant symptoms and changes including hot flashes, profuse sweating, headaches, increased weight, dryness and thinning of the vaginal walls, increased incidence of vaginal infections, depression, insomnia, loss of breast firmness, dizziness, sensations of cold in the hands and feet, irritability, pruritus of the sexual organs, constipation, artherosclerosis, and osteoporosis (Weideger, 1977). The widespread belief that all women experience the menopausal syndrome and that most experience this constellation of symptoms has lead to rather dramatic statements, such as "Menopause is not a temporary and passing period but a beginning of a progressive deterioration of a woman's body and mind" (Jern, 1973, p. x).

Several studies that report the results of surveys of large numbers of women of menopausal age have been published. McKinlay and Jeffreys (1974) sent a questionnaire to 638 women between the ages of 45 and 54. Hot flashes and night sweats were consistently associated with menopause and occurred in the majority of women; headaches, dizzy spells, palpitations, sleeplessness, depression, and weight increase showed no direct relationship to the menopause and were reported by 30 to 50% of the sample. In a later postal survey by Ballinger (1975, 1976), 539 women between the ages of 40 and 55 were sent a questionnaire that was intended to assess depressive and neurotic illness. Subjects were categorized according to premenopausal, menopausal, early postmenopausal, and late post-menopausal status; the data were also analyzed according to age categories regardless of menopausal status. The only significant difference was that women between the ages of 45 and 49 who were premenopausal had more psychiatric problems than premenopausal women between the ages of 40 to 44. The author interpreted his data to imply that there is a rise in psychiatric morbidity before the menopause that does not persist beyond one year past menopause but that vasomotor symptoms such as hot flashes and night sweats seem clearly related to the menopausal years. Finally, Chakravarti and colleagues (1977) surveyed women who had had a bilateral oophorectomy. Vasomotor symptoms were the most common problem reported, followed by depression and sexual dysfunction in the form of loss of libido or dyspareunia. Thus, surveys of symptoms in menopausal women have not consistently supported the existence of the traditional menopausal syndrome.

Similar conclusions were reached in a factor analytic study of climacteric symptoms by Greene (1976). He sampled 50 women between the ages of 40 to 55 who had complained of vasomotor and other symptoms. All completed a 30-item symptom scale in which they indicated the extent of each symptom. Three factors emerged from the factor analysis that accounted for 38% of the variance: a psychological factor, which included fatigue, worrying, tension, depression, panic attacks, disturbed sleep, excitability, crying; a somatic factor, which included dizziness, numbness or tingling, weight gain, headaches, blind spots in the vision, feelings of suffocation; and a vasomotor factor, which included hot flashes, sweating, and cold hands and feet. The labeling of the first two factors appears rather arbitrary, since, for example, fatigue could be viewed as a somatic symptom and feelings of suffocation could better be considered a psychological symptom. However, of primary interest was the fact that the factors were not significantly correlated—that is, suffering from symptoms in one category was not related to the probability that the woman would suffer symptoms from another category—again suggesting that the "menopausal syndrome" may not be a valid concept, since "syndrome" is typically used to refer to a group of symptoms that tend to occur together.

One difficulty in the interpretation of such research has been the lack of a reliable and valid measure of menopausal symptoms. One measure was developed by Kupperman and coworkers (1953); the Menopausal Index consists of 11 symptoms—vasomotor complaints, paresthesia, insomnia, nervousness, melancholia, vertigo, weakness or fatigue, arthralgia and myalgia, headaches, palpitations, and formication—the latter being a form of paresthesia in which there is a sensation as of ants running over the skin. In determining a person's score on the index, symptoms are weighted differently, with vasomotor symptoms being given a weight of "4," paresthesia, insomnia, and nervousness a weight of "2," and all others a weight of "1," although the authors do not offer a justification for the differential weighting system. There are no reliability data available for the scale, and there has been no assessment of the validity of the scale as a measure of menopausal symptoms.

The Biomedical Model
of Menopausal Symptoms

The primary theoretical model for conceptualizing menopausal symptoms has been a biomedical one; it states that both physical and psychological symptoms are the direct result of estrogen withdrawal or the result of biochemical changes that result from estrogen withdrawal such as the elevated gonadotropin levels found in menopausal women. Relevant to the evaluation of this model are studies assessing the covariation between symptoms and hormonal levels. Abe and colleagues (1977) assessed serum levels of estradiol, progesterone, FSH, and LH in 191 premenopausal and postmenopausal women and correlated hormonal levels with symptom severity as measured by Kupperman's Menopausal Index; none of the correlations was significant for the women who were experiencing menopause. Similar results were found in a group of women tested after bilateral ovariectomy; those who experienced vasomotor symptoms did not differ in blood levels of estrogen, LH, or FSH from those who did not experience symptoms (Aksel et al., 1976). On the other hand, Hutton and coworkers (1978) measured plasma levels of estrone and estradiol at 20- to 30-minute intervals for up to 24 hours in postmenopausal or ovariectomized women and compared hormonal levels of groups of women categorized according to symptoms; women with superficial dyspareunia and women with both dyspareunia and vasomotor symptoms had significantly lower levels of estradiol, but not of estrone, than women with only hot flashes and those who were symptom-free.

Indirect evidence related to the etiology of menopausal symptoms comes from studies that have tested the effects of exogenous estrogen on menopausal symptoms. As early as 1950, Fessler noted that hormonal treatment was effective in relieving hot flashes, but not irritability and depression. Kaufman (1967) found that hot flashes and atrophic vaginitis were successfully treated with hormones in close to 100% of the women, while only about 50% experienced relief from common emotional symptoms. In the evaluation of this type of research, improvement due to expectation must be considered; therefore, the effects of exogenous estrogen should be compared to the effects of placebos in a design in which neither the subjects nor the evaluators are aware of which compound the woman has been given. Only in this way can one evaluate the pharmacological effects of the active treatment.

A treatment study satisfying these criteria was reported by Utian (1972) who evaluated the effectiveness of exogenous estrogen treatment on various menopausal symptoms by comparing estrogen to placebo treatment in women with natural and surgical menopause. Only hot flashes and atrophic vaginitis were relieved by estrogen, but not by placebos, while symptoms of depression, irritability, insomnia, and palpitations responded significantly both to estrogen and to placebo therapy. The author concluded that these latter symptoms are, therefore, likely to be of psychological origin. Similar results have been found in several other studies that have employed a placebo control (George et al., 1973; Gerdes et al., 1982; Poller, Thomson, & Coope, 1980).

These studies do not strongly support the theory that most menopausal symptoms are due to hormonal changes. However, methodological problems, such as the lack of a reliable and valid measure of menopausal symptoms and the relatively small number of studies, preclude any definitive conclusions at this time. Nevertheless, the research discussed above has lead theorists in this area to conclude that hot flashes and, perhaps, atrophic vaginitis are caused by the changing hormonal environment of menopause, while other somatic and psychological symptoms are the result of historical, cultural, and stress factors (Bart & Perlmutter, 1981; Christie Brown & Christie Brown, 1976; Dewhurst, 1976; Perlmutter, 1978; Rakoff, 1975).

Further Models
of Menopausal Symptoms

Other models of the etiology of menopausal symptoms include: (a) the "domino" theory, which postulates that hormonal factors cause hot flashes, while other symptoms such as insomnia, depression, and irritability are secondary to the hot flashes; (b) the premorbid personality model, which hypothesizes that psychological symptoms are an exacerbation of or a simple continuation of symptoms that existed prior to menopause; (c) the coincidental stress model, which suggests that the particular stresses that occur during the time of menopause, such as children leaving home or illness in or death of parents, predispose women to psychological problems; and (d) the cultural relativist model, which examines the effects of cross-cultural, societal, or historical factors, such as the influence of attitudes and stereotypes, on menopausal symptoms (Koeske, 1982).

The Premorbid Personality Model

The model in which some menopausal symptoms are viewed as being due to a history of poor adjustment rather than to the menopause has provided the theoretical context for several studies. In an early study by Donovan (1951), 110 women who had been referred for menopausal symptoms were extensively interviewed. In general, women with psychological complaints reported a lifelong history of similar complaints that obviously antedated the menopause. More recently, Polit and LaRocco (1980) received mailed questionnaires from 31 premenopausal women, 51 menopausal women, and 84 postmenopausal women. In addition to evaluating the typical menopausal symptoms, women also completed personality questionnaires. Menopausal psychological symptoms were found to be significantly associated with poor premorbid adjustment, while vasomotor symptoms and weight gain were less susceptible to the influence of personality variables. Bart and Grossman (1978) cited a study by Kraines reporting that women with a history of low self-esteem and little life satisfaction were those who had considerable difficulty with menopause. If one assumes that personality traits are relatively enduring characteristics, these data support the premorbid personality theory as a model for psychological symptoms. As Bart and Grossman (1978) have pointed out, "The menopause itself does not turn a healthy, functioning woman into an involutional psychotic" (p. 344).

The Coincidental Stress Model

Data from several studies indicate that stressful life events significantly contribute to the incidence and severity of psychological and

; during the menopausal years. Greene and Cooke [torn] ?y of 408 menopausal women, utilized Green's n factor analysis and described above, to evaluate)toms, and stressful life events were determined ′. Scores on both scales tended to rise in the late early 40s, decline a little in the late 40s and early off more sharply in the late 50s and early 60s.)wise multiple regression was employed, with symptoms being the criterion variables and menopausal status, age, life stress, and the interactions among these variables being the predictors. The contribution of life stress was significant for both psychological and somatic symptoms and accounted for 38% and 43% of the variance in psychological and somatic symptoms, respectively. A significant interaction suggested that the relationship between symptoms and stress was greater in younger than in older women. The contribution of menopausal status in accounting for the variance in symptomatology was small and nonsignificant.

In a reanalysis of the data from the same sample, Cooke and Greene (1981) divided the stressful life events into those that involved "exit" events such as a child leaving home or the death of a family member or close friend, and other miscellaneous stressors. In a stepwise regression analysis, they found that miscellaneous stressors accounted for 39% of the variance in psychological symptoms, while a combination of exit events and miscellaneous events accounted for 40% of the variance in somatic symptoms; women with high scores on only one type of stressor and women scoring low on both reported few symptoms. They also pointed out that women between the ages of 35 and 54 experienced the most stress, and that almost all of this stress was due to exit events, with 60% due to deaths. These studies suggest that stress is a major contributing factor in the psychological and somatic symptoms of menopause and that stressful life events are more likely to occur during the years before, during, and after menopause. Unfortunately, in neither study did the authors report the relationship between stress and scores on the vasomotor factor of their scale.

In the studies on the relationship between stress and menopausal symptoms, the symptoms of major interest have been psychological and psychosomatic. There seems to have been an implicit assumption that hot flashes and atrophic vaginitis are caused by hormonal changes associated with menopause. Evidence from a variety of sources points to the validity of this assumption; however, although the primary cause of hot flashes and atrophic vaginitis may be hormonal, it is possible that stress exacerbates either the intensity of these symptoms and/or the woman's ability to cope with them. Unfortunately, there is little data on the effects of stress on these symptoms.

The Cultural Relativist Model

Koeske's (1982) cultural relativist model ". . . seeks to identify societal values or social, political, or economic factors which influence cultural stereotypes of the menopause" (p. 7). According to this model, women's roles in Western society, and particularly in the United States, are limited not only in number, and not only to roles of relatively low status but also to primarily biological roles. Women in our society are evaluated with regard to their biological capacity for being attractive and bearing and raising children, while for men biology is less important than is performance and intellect (Osofsky & Seidenberg, 1970). Given such culturally defined roles, it is not surprising that women view menopause negatively and that they experience adverse psychological consequences when they are no longer capable of fulfilling the major roles available to them. A parallel situation for men might be the depression, tension, and irritability experienced upon retirement—a time when they experience a loss of significant roles.

To appreciate more fully the influence of cultural values and stereotypes on the experience of menopause, one may consider the similarities and dissimilarities among menopause, pregnancy, and puberty. All three are natural events in women's lives, all three involve dramatic hormonal changes, and all three are associated with psychological and behavioral changes. However, the discomfort or pain of pregnancy is taken in stride and the psychological and behavioral quirks of pregnancy are met with understanding and indulgence, while the difficulties of menopause are viewed as signs of deterioration and the menopausal woman as pathetic (Weideger, 1977).

Although empirical support for a cultural model of menopausal symptoms is scarce, some research has investigated certain assumptions implicit in such a model. First, if the type and severity of symptoms are culturally determined, then this effect is most probably mediated by attitudes toward menopause. Frey (1982) evaluated attitudes toward menopause in a community sample and reported that professional women were more likely to have a wellness-orientation toward menopause (as opposed to having an illness-orientation) than were blue-collar woman workers and that, in general, employed women had fewer menopausal symptoms than did unemployed women. In a cross-cultural comparison, Vara (1970) notes that Finnish women are far less likely to experience menopausal symptoms than are American women and attributes this difference to the fact that Finnish women view menopause as a natural process, while American women view menopause as an unavoidable illness. Such correlational research on the relationship between attitudes toward menopause and symptoms of menopause, although relevant, suffers from interpretational problems; these data are frequently considered support for the hypothesis that attitudes influence symptoms, but just as logical is the conclusion that women who experience symptoms will develop a negative attitude toward menopause.

A second assumption of the cultural model is that attitudes and symptoms will vary across cultures. Bart (1969) examined ethnographic material from six societies—three in which women's status went up at midlife, one in which it remained the same, and two in which it went down. In societies where aging increased one's status and perceived wisdom, where the desexualization associated with menopause made women less threatening to men, or where women's freedom increased with menopause, there was little evidence of psychological and emotional difficulties associated with menopause. On the other hand, in Samoa, where most of the heavy work on plantations is done by women aged between 45 and 55, menopause was marked by temporary instability, food finickiness, and whims. Similar results were reported by Flint (1975), who studied 483 Indian women from a society in which premenopausal women were forbidden certain activities because they were viewed as contaminative, while menopausal women were allowed considerably more freedom. These women exhibited very few problems with menopause and offered no complaints of depression or incapacitation.

Maoz and colleagues (1970) conducted individual interviews with 55 middle-aged women; the interview material was evaluated for positive attitudes such as freedom from menstruation and pregnancy and a sense of liberation and negative attitudes such as loss of fertility, poor health, loss of femininity and youth, and fear of emotional and somatic disturbance. Only 21% of the European subjects expressed primarily positive attitudes, while 52% of the Orientals were so categorized. Consistent with these results is an anecdotal note by Weideger (1977), who quotes a psychiatrist working in China who said she had never seen a menopausal psychosis in a Chinese woman; this she attributed to the secure and coveted position of elderly women in China.

These studies suggest that in cultures where menopause is associated with a loss of significant roles and a reduction in power and freedom, the primary societal attitude toward menopause will be negative and menopausal women will experience adverse psychological consequences. In our society, although the picture is currently changing, the primary roles allowed to women have been those of child-bearing and child-rearing, and women with youth and beauty have been more valued than those with wisdom and experience. Thus, it is not surprising that many menopausal women experience depression and anxiety during the menopausal years, nor is it surprising that such symptoms are not relieved with hormone medication.

A third assumption implicit in the cultural model is that attitudes toward menopause and symptoms of menopause vary among distinct subgroups within a culture. Bart (1971) conducted extensive interviews with 20 middle-aged women hospitalized for depression. She reported that women who had overprotective and overinvolved relationships with their children were more likely to experience menopausal depression than those without such relationships and that housewives had a higher rate of depression than working women. The conclusion that employed women are less likely to suffer from menopausal depression has been supported by several other studies (Frey, 1982; Polit & LaRocco, 1980). Severne (1982) interviewed 922 Belgian women between the ages of 46 and 55. While hot flashes were relatively independent of employment status and social class, psychological symptoms (insomnia, nervousness, irritability, headaches, and depression) were related to both variables. Lower socioeconomic status (SES) subjects with a job had the most pronounced symptoms, while symptoms were virtually nonexistent for higher SES subjects with a job. The author suggests that employment does not protect the lower SES women since their work is probably unstimulating but physically more demanding.

Dege and Gretzinger (1982) assessed attitudes toward menopause in men and women with different levels of education and found that the more educated subjects, both men and women, had more positive attitudes toward menopause than did the less educated subjects. The results of these studies are theoretically consistent with the cultural model, since one would expect that, compared to unemployed and/or uneducated women, employed and/or educated women would be less likely to rely exclusively on biological roles for their self-esteem but would attribute importance to other roles related to their work and their intellect.

Although the studies presented above support cultural factors as being etiological in menopausal symptoms, Koeske (1982) argues for considering such factors in the context of interacting with other influences.

> It is important to acknowledge that sociocultural factors also influence the actual levels of important biological variables, thereby indirectly influencing bodily experience and behavior: gene pools, diet, exercise, obesity, sleep, physical and emotional stress, parity, lactation, disease history, available medical care—all are influenced by social and cultural factors in complex and probably unknown ways. The estrogen decline that comes with increasing age may not be associated with identical body changes and body experiences when the accompanying physiological context varies. Thus, such characteristics of the menopause as age at last menstrual period, length of perimenopause, pattern of endocrine–hormone changes, and types of patterns of associated body changes may covary with such factors as obesity, current and lifetime stress, speed of role loss or role change, current diet, exercise, or sleep patterns, and pre-existing disease states or propensities. And influences such as these will in part reflect the operation of sociocultural factors that have been translated into a lifetime of multiple influences (p. 12).

Summary

In conclusion, there are a variety of different conceptual models that aid our understanding of menopausal symptoms and within which we can attempt to integrate divergent information. It is probable that no one model is sufficient, and all are necessary to explain the complex experience of menopause. Nevertheless, some tentative conclusions can be drawn. Symptoms of menopause should, perhaps, be separated into two distinct types: one category for physical symptoms, consisting of vasomotor symptoms and atrophic vaginitis; a second category for psychological symptoms, consisting of fatigue, depression, tension, insomnia, irritability, headaches, and weight gain. Support for such a distinction is found within the context of every model discussed in this section. Psychological symptoms seem to be unrelated to hormonal levels but do seem to covary with premenopausal personality characteristics, levels of stress, and cultural factors, while physical symptoms tend to covary somewhat with hormonal levels and seem unrelated to personality, stress, or cultural factors. All may be considered "menopausal symptoms" in the sense that all may be complaints of women experiencing menopause and in the sense that menopause is a psychological, cultural, and physiological event.

13

The Menopausal Hot Flash

The most common complaints of menopausal women are those associated with vasomotor instability. Hot flashes, characterized by sensations of heat, usually in the face, neck, and chest and sometimes followed by perspiration and/or shivering, are frequently noticed prior to the complete cessation of menses and continue in the early years after menopause. They seem to be most frequent and most intense shortly after cessation of menses and shortly after surgery in women having bilateral oophorectomy. There is surprisingly little reliable information on the percentage of women who experience hot flashes during menopause or on the length of time the symptom persists, although it has been assumed that this symptom occurs in the majority of women and that, without treatment, hot flashes abate over time and eventually cease completely. Women seeking medical help for hot flashes are typically placed on hormone replacement therapy (HRT) consisting of estrogen or a combination of estrogen and progesterone—both of which tend to alleviate the symptoms.

In the only published descriptive study of the menopausal hot flash, Voda (1982) had 20 menopausal women keep records of their hot flashes for two weeks. She presented the following summary information based on 912 hot flash records: the mean duration was 3.31 minutes; of the 912, 534 started in the neck, head, scalp, and ears, 68 in the neck and/or breasts, 59 below the breasts, 19 in the neck and above the breasts, 118 in the breasts and/or below the breasts, and 114 all over; the direction of spread varied, some up, some down, some both; the time of day or night varied, with no particular time for the majority; and there did not seem to be a common trigger such as eating or stress.

Physiological Concomitants of Hot Flashes

Until recently, the only information on hot flashes was based on self-report data. However, during the past several years, attempts have been made to develop objective indices of hot flashes. The most obvious measure of the symptom is body temperature, although researchers have also found changes in other physiological variables to be associated with the occurrence of hot flashes. One of the first studies was reported by Meldrum and colleagues (1979). They recorded finger temperature for eight hours in seven women who were within two years of surgical or natural menopause and who were experiencing frequent hot flashes; the women were asked to report all subjective feelings of flushing in the recording session. There were 41 significant (1°C) elevations in finger temperature, 28 of which coincided with subjectively reported hot flashes; for these 28, the mean duration of the skin temperature elevation was 31 minutes, and the duration of the subjective sensation was 2.3 minutes. The subjective sensation began an average of 1.2 minutes before and ended 1.1 minutes after the onset of the temperature increase. (The typical temporal relationship between finger temperature and subjective hot flashes is depicted in Figure 13.1.) Five of these subjects received HRT for one to three months and were reassessed; there was a significant reduction in the number of temperature elevations.

Tataryn and coworkers (1981) studied eight postmenopausal women with frequent and severe hot flashes for 8 or 16 hours, during which time continuous recordings of finger temperature, skin conductance, and core temperature—measured in the external auditory meatus—were taken. They consistently found the first change to be an increase in skin conductance, followed by a rise in finger temperature, then followed by a decrease in core

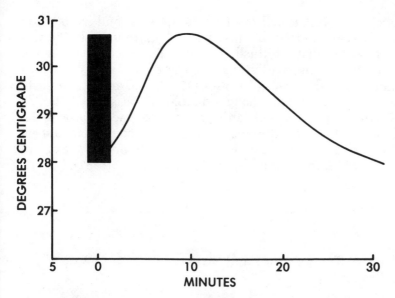

Figure 13.1. Mean characteristics and typical configuration of finger temperature fluctuations associated with hot flashes. The shaded area delineates the period from the mean beginning to completion of subjective flushing.

Reprinted by permission of the C. V. Mosby Company from D. R. Meldrum, I. M. Shamonki, A. M. Frumar, I. V. Tataryn, R. J. Chang, and H. L. Judd. "Elevations in skin temperature of the finger as an objective index of postmenopausal hot flashes: Standardization of the technique." American Journal of Obstetrics and Gynecology, 1979, 135, 713-17.

temperature. Of the subjectively reported flashes, 82%, 98%, and 81% were associated with changes in finger temperature, skin conductance, and core temperature, respectively, and 76% were associated with changes in all three. Four women were reassessed after one month of HRT, and there was a significant reduction in both the subjective sensations and the frequency and magnitude of the finger temperature changes.

Cardiovascular responses associated with hot flashes were measured by Ginsburg. Swinhoe, and O'Reilly (1981) in six women. The first circulatory change was a rapid rise in hand blood flow, which, in some patients, occurred before the subjective sensation. Hand flow increased in each instance of a subjectively reported flash and remained elevated for an average of 2.5 minutes; there was a lesser increase in forearm blood flow.

Subjective sensations lasted from 1 to 5 minutes, and hand blood flow usually remained elevated for at least a minute after the woman had reported that the flush was over. There was a significant increase in heart rate, which occurred after the subjective sensation and returned to control values prior to the end of the flash; there were no significant changes in blood pressure. Although these data indicate consistent cardiovascular changes to be associated with hot flashes, finger temperature and skin conductance seem to be the more popular measures for objectively documenting hot flashes (Erlik, Meldrum, & Judd, 1982; Laufer et al., 1982).

The Effects of Temperature and Stress on Hot Flashes

There has been some research attention directed at the effects of environmental variables, activity, and stress on hot flashes. Molnar (1981) found a correlation of .68 between the number of flashes per day and outdoor temperature, while Voda (1981) found no relationship between ambient temperature and frequency of hot flashes but did report hot flashes to be of longer duration in hot weather than in cooler weather.

An underlying assumption apparent in the literature is that hot flashes increase in frequency or duration under periods of emotional stress, but empirical support for such a relationship is lacking. Rogers (1956) and Friederich (1982), in their reviews of menopausal symptoms, state that hot flashes occur more often at times of emotional stress but cite no supporting references. Ginsburg, Swinhoe, and O'Reilly (1981) wished to measure physiological changes that accompany hot flashes. To the women in their study who did not have spontaneous hot flashes during the recording session, they gave mental arithmetic problems; they justified this procedure by stating that the stress of the problems would induce hot flashes. Unfortunately, they did not report whether this procedure was effective. Since stress has been found to be related to a variety of physical and psychological symptoms, a potentially productive area of research would be the study of the relationship between hot flashes and stress; such studies are currently being conducted in my laboratory.

Etiology of Hot Flashes

Estrogen

Originally, it was thought that declining levels of estrogen due to ovarian failure at the time of menopause were the cause of hot flashes. Such a belief has been bolstered by the fact that exogenous estrogen alleviates hot flashes in the majority of menopausal women who suffer from them. However, research during the last ten years has not been supportive of this theory. Aksel and coworkers (1976) assessed plasma estrogen levels and vasomotor symptoms in 22 women undergoing bilateral oophorectomy. Estrogen fell on the second day after surgery, and approximately one-third developed hot flashes prior to leaving the hospital; plasma estrogen levels were similar in women with and without symptoms. More recently, Hutton and colleagues (1978) determined plasma levels of estrone and estradiol at 20- to 30-minute intervals for up to 24 hours in 26 postmenopausal or ovariectomized women. Women experiencing hot flashes did not have lower estrogen levels than those not experiencing hot flashes, and there was no obvious relationship between the timing of a flash and estrogen level or change in estrogen level during the 24 hours.

On the other hand, the most recent study in this area (Erlik, Meldrum, & Judd, 1982) did find estrogen levels to be related to hot flashes. They tested 24 postmenopausal women who reported at least 12 hot flashes per day and 24 who had never experienced the symptom. Blood was sampled four times at 15-minute intervals. Mean age, body weight, percentage of ideal weight, total estrone and estradiol, and the percentage of non-bound estradiol were significantly lower in symptomatic women than in symptom-free women. Since symptom-free women were heavier, the higher estrogen levels in these women may have been due to the ability of adipose tissue to aromatize androgens to estrogens (Frisch, Canick & Tulchinsky, 1980). Estrogens produced in this way may act to reduce vasomotor symptoms in the same way that exogenous estrogen does. Although these data may be interpreted as support for the theory that hot flashes are caused by lowered estrogen levels, other interpretations are possible. The possibility exists that estrogen may alleviate vasomotor symptoms but that the lack of estrogen does not cause such symptoms. Indeed, several researchers in this area (Maddock, 1978; Casper, Yen, & Wilkes, 1979) have argued against lowered estrogen levels as the cause of menopausal hot flashes since other conditions characterized by low levels of estrogen, such as primary gonadal failure and gonadal dysgenesis, or by rapidly falling levels of estrogen, such as during the premenstrual phase or prior to labor, are not typically associated with hot flashes.

Luteinizing Hormone

Another theory concerned with the etiology of menopausal hot flashes hypothesizes that the cause lies in the elevated levels of or in the increased pulsatile amplitude of LH that occurs during menopause. In the study by Aksel and coworkers (1976) described above, plasma levels of LH in women experiencing hot flashes following oophorectomy were similar to those who were symptom-free. More damaging to the LH theory are two studies reporting hot flashes in women with low levels of LH. Mulley, Mitchell, and Tattersal (1977) described two patients who experienced hot flashes after surgical removal of the pituitary. Similarly, Meldrum and coworkers (1981b) studied two women with pituitary insufficiency. In both, LH levels were low compared to premenopausal women, and the relationships of finger temperature and skin conductance to subjectively reported flashes were identical to that of the typical postmenopausal flush. These women did, however, exhibit LH pulses of low amplitude in a close temporal association with the finger temperature rise.

Although hot flashes seem unrelated to LH levels, support for a temporal association with LH pulses is provided by Tataryn and colleagues (1979). Six postmenopausal women who suffered from frequent hot flashes were studied for eight continuous hours. Finger temperature was recorded; blood samples were taken every 15 minutes, and every 5 minutes during subjectively reported flashes. Thirty-four temperature changes of at least 1°C were identified; 32 of these were subjectively reported. There were 31 LH pulses, and 26 of these pulses occurred simultaneously with a temperature rise. (Data from one woman is presented in Figure 13.2.) The peak of the LH pulse occurred, on the average, 13.7 minutes after the onset of the temperature increase and 7.4 minutes after the peaking of skin temperature. Similarly, Meldrum and coworkers (1980) recorded finger temperature continuously for eight hours and drew blood samples in six postmenopausal women. LH changes were significantly correlated with finger temperature, and LH peaked 5 to 10 minutes after the onset of the finger temperature increase. Finally,

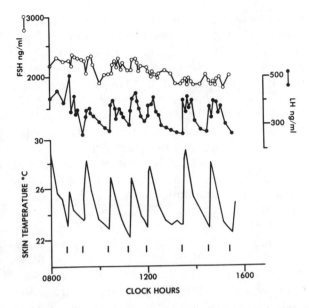

Figure 13.2. Changes in cutaneous finger temperature, serum LH, and FSH levels over eight hours in a postmenopausal woman. Note the close temporal relationship between each subjective hot flash (indicated by vertical bars), temperature elevations, and pulses of LH release.

Reprinted by permission from I. V. Tataryn, D. R. Meldrum, K. H. Lu, A. M. Frumar, and H. L. Judd. "LH, FSH, and skin temperature during the menopausal hot flash." *Journal of Clinical Endocrinology and Metabolism,* 1979, 49, 152–54.

Lightman and colleagues (1981) found significant increases in LH, which occurred after the flush. Thus, although LH pulses and hot flashes tend to be temporally associated in postmenopausal women, the specific relationship argues against the LH pulse as being etiological in the hot flash.

Gonadotropin-Releasing Hormone

The temporal relationships discussed above indicate that the hot flash may be caused by some mechanism that induces both an LH pulse and the subjective feeling of a hot flash. A logical candidate for such a mechanism is the hypothalamic release of GnRH, as evidenced by elevated GnRH levels during postmenopause. Data on

GnRH levels in postmenopausal women, presented in a previous section, is contradictory, and GnRH has been found to range from being virtually undetectable to being significantly higher than those found in premenopausal women. No conclusions can be drawn from these studies, since the typical methodology of sampling blood at regular intervals is not appropriate for evaluating levels of a substance that is released episodically, as is the case with GnRH.

Another theoretical explanation for the temporal, but not causal, relationship between LH pulses and hot flashes is the coincidental anatomic proximity between GnRH-secreting neurons and the thermoregulatory center. Meldrum and coworkers (1981b) have speculated that "Some of the hypothalamic neurons which contain GnRH and the preoptic/anterior hypothalamic nuclei that regulate body temperature are in a close anatomic relationship, suggesting that neurotransmitter signals associated with GnRH release may modify thermoregulating neurons and trigger a hot flash" (p. 686). This theory is endorsed by Laufer and colleagues (1982), who successfully treated hot flashes with clonidine, an alpha-adrenergic receptor agonist that stimulates alpha receptors in the depression site of the vasomotor center of the medulla oblongata. They suggest that clonidine constituted effective treatment because it inhibited catecholamine-induced stimulation in the thermoregulatory center and in the hypothalamic neurons containing GnRH—the latter being a coincidental effect due to the proximity of the two areas and not related to the treatment effectiveness. Interestingly, Tulandi, Lal, and Kinch (1983) reported that clonidine effected improvement in the subjective report of vasomotor symptoms, but LH pulses and levels were unaffected.

Clayden, Bell, and Pollard (1974) have also found clonidine successful in treatment for hot flashes; however, their rationale for clonidine treatment was that this drug, which has been successfully used to treat persons with migraine headaches, diminishes vascular reactivity. Voda (1982), in her study of 20 menopausal women with hot flashes, noted that all complained of previously having experienced premenstrual headaches, and eight reported a long-standing history of premenopausal migraine headaches occurring during the premenstruum. Voda speculated that women who experience hot flashes during the menopause may be those with a predisposition either for thermoregulatory problems, or for vascular instability, or for both. Since premenstrual migraines and menopausal hot flashes are both associated with falling levels of estrogen, it is tempting to speculate that estrogen levels are associated with hot flashes by influencing vascular reactivity. Although provocative, the theory proposed here is complex and, in order to aid in the understanding and treatment of hot flashes, requires elaboration and empirical validation.

In summary, the cause of menopausal hot flashes is, as yet, unknown. Lowered estrogen levels, LH pulses, and skin conductance changes are associated with hot flashes, but there is no empirical support for a causal relationship. Elevated levels or increased pulse amplitudes of GnRH are a possible causal agent but are, as yet, unverified. Research during the last decade, however, is encouraging in that hot flashes, previously considered of insufficient consequence to merit serious investigation, are the subject of an increasing number of studies, and improved methodologies for the investigation of hot flashes are being developed.

14

Osteoporosis

Osteoporosis is characterized by a decrease in skeletal mass or quantity of bone, without a change in the quality of the existing bone. New bone is continually formed and existing bone continually resorbed throughout life, but peak bone mass is reached at about age 30 to 35, after which time bone resorption exceeds bone formation, and all persons lose bone with advancing age. This reduction in bone mass is regarded as the major factor in osteoporotic fractures, which typically occur in the vertebra, distal radius, and the hips. The rate of bone loss varies among individuals, and those with high rates of bone loss and demonstrated susceptibility to fractures are viewed as suffering from osteoporosis. It is generally believed that menopause is at least a contributory factor, and possibly the primary factor, in the development of osteoporosis. Although there are no reliable statistics regarding the percentage of menopausal women who suffer from this disorder, the incidence is believed to be considerably less than the incidence for other symptoms such as hot flashes.

Bone metabolism is a complex process and dependent upon a variety of interacting systems for normal activity. Calcium is a crucial ingredient in the making of bone and a by-product of bone absorption; intestinal absorption of calcium from the diet is the primary source of calcium, and vitamin D is essential for adequate calcium absorption. Vitamin D is converted to its active form, 1,25-dihydroxyvitamin D, in the kidneys, and this conversion is dependent upon adequate levels of parathyroid hormone (PTH). PTH is, thus, a primary factor in the regulation of serum calcium levels. Increases in PTH, which can be triggered by falling levels of calcium, cause an accelerated rate of bone resorption and an increase in serum and urinary calcium. Calcitonin, a hormone secreted by the thyroid, has effects opposite those of PTH and decreases the rate of bone remodeling.

Since osteoporosis is characterized by a decrease in skeletal mass, a variety of biochemical measures, such as high serum and urinary concentrations of calcium, low levels of 1,25-dihydroxyvitamin D, high levels of PTH, and/or low levels of calcitonin as well as direct measures of intestinal absorption of calcium using radioactive isotopes have been viewed as positive indications of this disorder. Similarly, there are a variety of measures that are assumed to reflect bone health, such as bone density, bone size, bone mineral content, and/or fractures. Given such a wide array of potential variables to study, methodological variation in research on osteoporosis is considerable, and, as might be expected, the results are somewhat contradictory.

The Effects of Menopause, Estrogen, and Aging on Osteoporosis

Those who consider osteoporosis to be a menopausal symptom assume that the decreasing levels of estrogen associated with menopause are responsible for osteoporosis in women (Gallagher & Nordin, 1974). Young and Nordin (1967) assessed plasma and urinary levels of calcium and phosphorus, which they assumed would be elevated in individuals with an increased rate of bone resorption, in premenopausal and postmenopausal women and found postmenopausal women to have elevated levels of calcium and phosporus. These date are suggestive of the etiological nature of menopause in osteoporosis and are consistent with the results of a recent study (Frumar et al., 1980), which found the urinary calcium to creatinine ratio (Ca:Cr), an index of bone resorption, to be significantly and negatively correlated with plasma estrogen in postmenopausal women.

On the other hand, since bone loss is a natural process of aging and since menopause occurs at a similar age in most women, it has been difficult to differentiate the effects of menopause from those of aging on the osteoporotic process. Bullamore and colleagues (1970) measured calcium absorption by plasma radioactivity after ingestion of oral calcium isotopes in men and women between the ages of 20 and 95. Absorption of calcium fell with age after 60 years of age, and everyone over 80 had significant malabsorption. Since deficits in the intestinal absorption of calcium have been assumed to be one possible factor in osteoporosis, the authors concluded that this malabsorption of calcium associated with the aging process may be etiological in osteoporosis.

In order to differentiate those effects on bone loss due to aging from those due to menopause, several studies have evaluated bone loss in women who had had bilateral oophorectomy prior to menopause. Aitken and coworkers (1973) compared whole-bone density in women who had had a hysterectomy to those who had had a hysterectomy and bilateral oophorectomy. Neither type of surgery influenced bone density if the woman was over 45 at the time of the surgery. In women who had surgery before the age of 45, the oophorectomized group had significantly lower values of bone density measured six years post-surgery than did women who had had only hysterectomy. In a similar study, Lindsay and colleagues (1978) found oophorectomized women to have significantly less bone density than hysterectomized women three years post-surgery. They estimated the loss of bone mineral to be approximately 2% per year in the years immediately following oophorectomy, then a decrease to 0.8% per year, while women experiencing natural menopause exhibited a loss of 1% per year.

Since the subjects in these studies were not selected on the basis of the presence or absence of osteoporosis, we do not know how many of the subjects actually suffered from this disorder. Positive indications of osteoporosis are more likely at advanced age, menopausal status is correlated with age, the probability of a woman having had a bilateral oophorectomy is correlated with age, and not all postmenopausal women exhibit signs of osteoporosis. The independent contribution of menopause, natural or surgical, to the etiology of osteoporosis has been difficult to establish.

In an effort to address this issue and to evaluate the assumption that, if bone loss does increase after menopause or the surgical loss of the ovaries, this loss is due to the decreased levels of estrogen, researchers have compared osteoporotic women to normal postmenopausal women on levels of sex steroids. Davidson and coworkers (1982) found postmenopausal fracture patients to have a lower percentage of ideal weight and significantly higher concentrations of sex-hormone-binding globulin (SHBG), resulting in lower concentrations of biologically active estradiol and testosterone, than did postmenopausal women without fractures. In contrast, two studies compared hormone levels in postmenopausal women with vertebral crush fractures to age-matched controls: Riggs and colleagues (1973) found no group differences in plasma testosterone, serum estrogen, or serum gonadotropins; Davidson and coworkers (1983) reported no group differences in cortisol, cortisol-binding globulin, testosterone, androstenedione, dehydroepiandrosterone, estrone, estradiol, or SHBG, but the fracture patients did have significantly lower spinal bone mineral density than did the controls. Riggs and colleagues (1973) concluded that some factor in addition to menopause causes the accelerated bone loss in osteoporotic patients.

The role of estrogen in bone metabolism has been investigated also with respect to changes associated with fluctuating estrogen levels during the normal menstrual cycle in premenopausal women. Baran and coworkers (1980) measured calcium, phosphate, parathyroid hormone, calcitonin, and 1,25-dihydroxyvitamin D on days 3 and 13 of the cycle in 12 women; no differences were noted in any of these variables, despite a three-fold difference in estradiol. In a recent study, Tjellegen and colleagues (1983) collected blood and urine samples every day for one cycle in five women; fluctuations in estradiol were indicative of normal ovulatory cycles. There were no significant changes associated with the cycle for 25-hydroxyvitamin D, 24,25-dihydroxyvitamin D, or serum calcium, but 1,25-dihydroxyvitamin D showed a significant midcycle peak, which the authors found difficult to interpret without corresponding changes in calcium metabolism.

The Effects
of Hormone Replacement Therapy
on Osteoporosis

Although the empirical evidence for low levels of estrogen being etiological in osteoporosis is weak, hormone replacement therapy (HRT) is frequently advocated, both as a treatment for osteoporosis and/or as a prophylactic. Research results have been relatively consistent in demonstrating improvement in parameters associated with osteoporosis in response to the administration of exogenous estrogen. Following estrogen treatment, improvement has been reported in serum calcium and phosphate (Moore et al., 1981), intestinal absorption of calcium (Caniggia et al., 1970), and the urinary calcium to creatinine ratio (Frumar et al., 1980; Geola et al., 1980;

Mandel et al., 1983). Dose–response relationships were noted by Christiansen and colleagues (1982); they administered high, medium, or low doses of estrogen to postmenopausal women and compared the results to a group receiving placebos. Bone mineral content declined by 2% in the placebo group, was unchanged in the low estrogen group, and increased by 0.8% and 1.5% in the medium and high groups, respectively.

Of perhaps greater importance are the effects of estrogen treatment on fractures. Nachtigall and colleagues (1979a) compared an untreated postmenopause group to a group of women who had received HRT for ten years and for whom the treatment had been begun within three years of menopause; there were seven fractures in the untreated group but none in the treated group. Jensen, Christiansen, and Transbol (1982) assessed the fracture frequency in groups receiving no HRT, short-term HRT, and long-term HRT; the number of women with postmenopausal fractures was 13% lower in the long-term treatment group than in the no-treatment group.

Others have noted that, although HRT may produce beneficial effects on osteoporosis in group comparisons, there is considerable individual variability in the response to estrogen (Lindsay et al., 1978). Gallagher, Riggs, and DeLuca (1980) compared the effects of placebo and estrogen treatment for six months on calcium absorption; the advantage of estrogen was demonstrated by a significant group increase in calcium absorption and in serum 1,25-dihydroxyvitamin D—both of which were unchanged with placebo. However, examination of individual data indicated such improvement in only seven of their twelve subjects. Factors related to individual differences in treatment response are suggested by Williams and coworkers (1982), who found that the benefits of HRT were greatest for thin women who also smoked. In obese nonsmokers, the risk neither of hip nor of forearm fractures was reduced by exogenous estrogen.

Researchers interested in the relationship between estrogen and osteoporosis have concentrated their efforts on the practical aspects—that is, the effects of HRT on indices of osteoporosis—but have neglected issues concerned with the processes that mediate these effects. Endogenous and exogenous estrogen levels may affect bone metabolism, but the mechanisms that mediate this effect have not been clarified. Hypothesized mechanisms include the following: estrogen may have direct effects on the osteoclasts or may exert effects by increasing calcitonin secretion or by increasing the sensitivity of bones to calcitonin (Aitken, 1976); it may inhibit bone resorption by inhibiting the effects of PTH on the bone (Nordin, 1971); it may increase calcium absorption via effects on vitamin D metabolism (Gallagher, Riggs, & DeLuca, 1980); it may reduce the responsiveness of the bone to PTH, reduce calcium loss through excretion, and increase the use of dietary calcium by increasing absorption (Nachtigall et al., 1979a); it may improve calcium balance by lowering fecal and urinary calcium (Gallagher & Nordin, 1974); or it may modify endogenous synthesis of 1,25-dihydroxyvitamin D or may enhance calcitonin secretion (Davidson et al., 1982).

Researchers (Young & Nordin, 1967; Davies, Mawer, & Adams, 1977) have pointed out that cause-and-effect relationships in osteoporosis need to be clarified because treatments such as estrogen may be modifying an effect rather than a cause of the disorder. For example, increases in bone resorption result in higher levels of calcium in the plasma, and estrogen may reduce plasma levels of calcium without actually decreasing the rate of bone reabsorption. Clearly, the magnitude and mechanism of the effect of menopause on bone metabolism and of the effect of exogenous estrogen treatment on osteoporosis have not, thus far, been delineated.

In conclusion, the studies discussed above suggest that osteoporosis may be a heterogenous disorder with regard to etiology and that low levels of estrogen may be regarded as one of many possible contributing factors. Consequently, the value of HRT in the treatment of osteoporosis is questionable. The research indicates that, to be of value, estrogen must be administered on a long-term basis and that treatment must be started soon after menopause and before any signs of osteoporosis appear. However, given that only a small percentage of postmenopausal women experience symptomatic osteoporosis, that estrogen is not beneficial to all women suffering from the disorder, that the mechanisms by which estrogen may be beneficial have not been clarified, and that long-term administration of exogenous estrogen is associated with an increased risk of uterine cancer, the recommendation that all women begin HRT at the time of menopause and continue on it indefinitely (Aitken, 1976; Gallagher & Nordin, 1974) does not reflect an unbiased consideration of the potential risks and benefits. Worley (1981) offers a recommendation more consistent with the empirical evidence— women in high-risk categories for osteoporosis, such as those who are thin, caucasian, smokers, related to women with postmenopausal osteoporosis, and/or inactive, should be offered HRT for the prevention of osteoporosis.

The Effects of Diet and Activity
on Osteoporosis

Studies investigating other biochemical factors in osteoporosis rein-
force the theory that this disorder has multiple causes. Hossain,
Smith, and Nordin (1970) took measures of the cortical area from
the second metacarpal in premenopausal and postmenopausal women who suffered either from hyperparathyroidism or from hypoparathyroidism. The rate of postmenopausal bone loss was reduced
in hypoparathyroidism and accelerated in hyperparathyroidism.
However, in a group of 16 women with postmenopausal osteoporosis, Teitelbaum and colleagues (1976) noted that only six had elevated levels of circulating parathyroid hormone. Low levels of estrogen are unlikely to be the sole determinant of parathyroid hormone
levels, since not all postmenopausal women exhibit elevated levels.
Interestingly, Muller (1969) has noted that in animals hyperparathyroidism can be induced by a prolonged phosphate-rich, calcium-
poor diet, again suggesting the interactive and heterogenous nature
of the disorder.

Another factor identified as influencing the probability of postmenopausal osteoporosis is weight. Williams and coworkers (1982)
noted that, in their sample of 929 women, the risk of osteoporosis
was 5 to 6 times greater in thin than in obese women. Similarly,
Frumar and colleagues (1980) found a significant negative correlation between the calcium to creatinine ratio and percent ideal
weight. As is discussed in detail elsewhere in this book, androgens
are converted to estrogen in adipose tissue, so obese women tend to
have higher levels of estrogen than thin women; thus, Nachtigall
and coworkers (1979a) have attributed the lowered incidence of
osteoporosis in obese women to their elevated levels of estrogen.
However, another explanation for these data is that increased body
weight places more stress on the bones, and bone is deposited in
proportion to the load that the bone must carry. Furthermore, according to the National Dairy Council (1982), the most important single
factor influencing fracture susceptibility is the peak bone mass
reached at maturity. Thus, an obese individual would be expected
to have a greater peak bone mass and to place more stress on their
bones—both factors would tend to increase the size and strength of
their bones in comparison to thinner women.

Diet is an obvious factor in osteoporosis, since calcium is
crucial to bone metabolism and our primary source of calcium is
diet. As noted above, Muller (1969) reported that prolonged phosphate-rich, calcium-poor diets in animals produced hyperpara-

thyroidism, which results in increased bone resorption and eventual deterioration of the bones. When calcium intake is inadequate, calcium is withdrawn from bone in order to maintain adequate plasma levels. The Recommended Daily Allowance of calcium is 800 mg, whereas according to the National Dairy Council (1982), 50% of U.S. women 15 years of age and older consume less than 600 mg/day, and 75% of women over the age of 35 have intakes below that recommended. In support of a dietary influence on the development of osteoporosis, these authors describe an epidemiological study in Yugoslavia in which groups were matched for ethnic origin, physical activity, and living conditions; the diet of one group contained 800 to 1,100 mg of calcium per day, while the diet of the other group contained 350 to 500 mg per day. Those with the higher calcium intake exhibited greater cortical bone density and reduced incidence of proximal femur fractures at all ages and for both sexes. The difference in bone mass was apparent at age 30, suggesting the importance of peak bone mass and calcium intake early in life as influencing the risk of fractures.

Since adequate calcium is obviously crucial to proper bone formation, calcium supplements and/or vitamin D, which is necessary for intestinal absorption of calcium, have been tested for their effects on osteoporosis. Riggs and colleagues (1976) administered 2.5 g of calcium and 400 units of vitamin D per day to one group of osteoporotic women and 2 g of calcium per day and 50,000 units of vitamin D twice a week to a second group. Both groups exhibited a significant decrease in bone resorbing surfaces, and the second group also showed a significant decrease in bone forming surfaces. Gallagher and Nordin (1974) reported results of a study comparing the effectiveness of calcium supplements and estrogen. Estrogen reduced metacarpal cortical bone loss from .044 mm/year to .007 mm/year; women on low-calcium diets lost .085 mm/year and those with calcium supplements lost .011 mm/year.

The effects of vitamin D have been assessed by Lawoyin and coworkers (1980), who administered a pharmacological dose of 25-hydroxyvitamin D to six women with osteoporosis for three months, which resulted in a significant increase in the intestinal absorption of calcium. Other studies have, however, cast doubt on the effectiveness of vitamin D therapy. Reeve and colleagues (1982) reported an immediate improvement in calcium absorption with 24,25-dihydroxyvitamin D, but this effect was lost after six months of treatment. Davies, Mawer, and Adams (1977) treated osteoporotic women with 1,25 dihydroxyvitamin D; the intestinal absorption of calcium was increased, but the calcium gained was excreted in the urine. Thus, the benefits of calcium and vitamin D treatment for osteoporosis have not been proven. It is surprising how little research has been devoted to such an obvious and safe treatment as calcium supplements or dietary changes in order to increase calcium intake and, ultimately, reduce the risk of osteoporosis. It should be noted that, because bone remodeling is a slow process, it may require up to two or three years for the effects of an increase in calcium intake to be evident (National Dairy Council, 1982).

An epidemiologic study by Smith and Rizek (1966) investigated the incidence of osteoporosis in women and its relation to a variety of interacting factors, such as race, diet, activity, socioeconomic status, and national origin. Two hundred Puerto Rican women and 2,063 Michigan women participated. Comparisons between the national groups revealed that the Puerto Ricans had a lower incidence of significant vertebral atrophy and a lower incidence of fractures than did the Michigan women. Interactive effects between country and race indicated that, for Michigan white women, the incidence of fractures increased linearly with age, while there were no vertebral crush fractures among Michigan blacks; similarly, among Puerto Ricans, only white women suffered from fractures. Whites and blacks both lost bone with age, but the rate was significantly less in black women than in white women (see Figure 14.1). Calcium intake was calculated in terms of milligrams per kilogram of body weight; Michigan whites consumed 15% less calcium than Michigan blacks, and all Puerto Ricans consumed 19% more calcium than did Michigan white women. Although physical activity was not measured directly, the socioeconomic class of the subjects implied probable differences. The Michigan white women were primarily middle-class and lead sedentary lives, while the Michigan blacks and the Puerto Ricans were from a lower SES class and had jobs that were more demanding physically. While assessing the independent contribution of these various factors to the development of osteoporosis was impossible due to experimental confounding, the results clearly implicate calcium intake and physical activity as possible contributors.

The effects of physical activity on bone formation in young persons is well established. Persons such as athletes, who engage in a regular exercise program, have heavier bones, and injuries that require immobilization of a limb result in bone becoming thin and decalcified. The fact that women begin to lose bone in their forties and men in their sixties has been interpreted as evidence for the influence of menopause and decreased estrogen levels on osteopo-

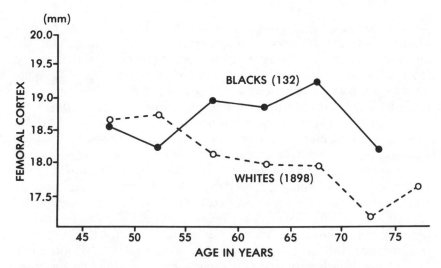

Figure 14.1. Mean values for femoral cortex in Michigan subjects by 5-year age groups.

Reprinted by permission of Lippincott/Harper & Row from R. W. Smith and J. Rizek. "Epidemiologic studies of osteoporosis in women of Puerto Rico and southeastern Michigan with special reference to age, race, national origin, and to other related or associated findings. *Clinical Orthopaedics,* 1966, 45, 31–48.

rosis in women (Gallaher & Nordin, 1974). However, the consequences of the traditional gender-related activities and careers promoted by our society—that of housewife for the woman and wage-earner for the man—are that a woman's career diminishes considerably when her children leave home, which usually occurs when a woman is in her 40s, and a man's career when he retires, which usually occurs when he is in his 60s. Both of these events may be accompanied by a drastic reduction in physical activity, which may contribute to osteoporosis. Cultural changes in the last decade of women pursuing careers and a strong emphasis on a regular exercise program for persons of both genders and all ages may decrease the incidence of osteoporosis in both men and women.

Summary

Osteoporosis is probably heterogenous in etiology and results from several interacting causes in any one individual. Considering osteoporosis a menopausal symptom is questionable, although the data seem to indicate that low levels of estrogen may contribute to the development of the disorder. However, such data are difficult to interpret since other factors that also appear to contribute to osteoporosis, such as a low-calcium diet or low levels of physical activity, have not been controlled for or measured in studies that have evaluated the influence of menopause on osteoporosis. Furthermore, given that menopause is a social and psychological, as well as a physiological, event, factors such as diet and physical activity may well covary with menopausal status. Research on the treatment of osteoporosis has been hampered by the widespread belief that insufficient estrogen is causal, and exogenous estrogen is a logical and effective treatment. Not only is the causal nature of estrogen and the treatment effectiveness of exogenous estrogen lacking in clear empirical support, but estrogen treatment is associated with the potential for serious, life-threatening side effects. Investigations on the treatment and/or prevention of osteoporosis with dietary improvements and/or increased levels of physical exercise constitute an exciting and potentially productive research endeavor.

15

The Treatment
of Menopausal Symptoms

Because of the widespread belief that the symptoms associated with menopause are due to lowered levels of estrogen, the most popular treatment for these symptoms has been and is exogenous estrogen or Hormone Replacement Therapy. By the 1940s, almost every major drug company offered some form of estrogen for the treatment of menopause. Although this treatment continues to be popular today, research during the past 20 years indicates that the benefits associated with HRT are less and the risks greater than was previously assumed, and, consequently, alternative forms of treatment are currently being investigated.

Hormone Replacement Therapy (HRT)

HRT and Vasomotor Symptoms

Vasomotor symptoms in the form of hot flashes and night sweats are undoubtedly the primary reason for menopausal women to seek medical help. The majority of women experience such symptoms to some degree, and for some women the symptoms are intense and disabling. Although there is little empirical evidence to support the theory that hot flashes are a manifestation of falling levels of estrogen, hormone replacement therapy (HRT) is the most common form of medical treatment for this symptom. Clinical trials of exogenous estrogen administration indicate that estrogen is, indeed, effective in relieving vasomotor symptoms in most women (Burnier et al., 1981; Hunter et al., 1977; Kaufman, 1967; Larsson-Cohn et al., 1978; Lind et al., 1979; Martin, Burnier, & Greaney, 1972; Reynolds et al., 1941). Furthermore, empirical studies in which estrogen therapy has been compared to placebos have consistently demonstrated estrogen to be superior to placebos in relieving vasomotor symptoms (Baumgardner et al., 1978; Coope, Thomson, & Pollner, 1975; Dennerstein et al., 1978; George et al., 1973; Lin et al., 1973; Poller, Thomson, & Coope, 1980; Utian, 1972).

Despite the success of this treatment, there are several unresolved issues concerning treatment of vasomotor symptoms with HRT that deserve further research consideration. Given the potential negative side effects of HRT (discussed below), it would be beneficial to patients to receive the minimal effective dose, and the dosage of estrogen necessary to relieve hot flashes completely or to an acceptable level has not been determined. Secondly, several authors (Archer, 1982; Voda, 1981) have expressed the belief that when HRT is stopped, vasomotor symptoms return, suggesting that estrogen only postpones the discomfort associated with these symptoms. Jeffcoate (1960) has suggested gradually reducing the dose of estrogen over a period of a few months in order to prevent the recurrence of vasomotor symptoms, but there is no empirical research to support this as a method of prevention.

this is ERT not HRT (which means estrogen + progestins)

HRT and Vaginal Symptoms

see p. 198

The only other menopausal symptom that appears to be treatable with estrogen is atrophic vaginitis. In postmenopause, the walls of the vagina become smooth and dry and produce less lubrication, and it has been assumed that this condition is due to a lack of estrogen. The karyopyknotic index (KPI), the percentage of superficial squamous cells with pyknotic nuclei (Morse et al., 1979), has become a popular method for determining, cytologically, the degree of estrogenicity of the vaginal smear, and the KPI has been found to be significantly correlated with plasma estradiol concentrations (Badawy et al., 1979; Morse et al., 1979). However, contradictory data have been reported by Lind and colleagues (1979) who noted that vaginal cytology is a poor indicator of estrogen status and by Kaufman (1967) who found little relationship between vaginal cytology, change in cytology, and severity of other symptoms. Two studies (Kupperman et al., 1953; Lin et al., 1973) found little or no relationship between improvement in vaginal cytology and improvement in other symptoms such as hot flashes.

Despite doubts concerning the relationship between circulating estrogen and objective measures of vaginal atrophy, estrogen is frequently prescribed to treat vaginal problems during menopause and postmenopause and is generally effective (Utian, 1972; Burnier et al., 1981). Although oral administration of estrogen has been found to produce a significant improvement in vaginal cytology when statistical analyses are applied to group data, Larsson-Cohn and colleagues (1978) noted that 40% of their subjects exhibited no change, and Geola and coworkers (1980) found that only a relatively high dose of oral estrogen improved the KPI to premenopausal values. On the other hand, vaginal administration of estrogen has been found more consistently to be effective in relieving the symptoms of atrophic vaginitis (Bercovici, Uretzki, & Patti, 1972; Deutsch, Ossowski, & Benjamin, 1981). Mandel and colleagues (1983) have reported that quite small doses of conjugated equine estrogens (.3 mg/day) administered vaginally returned vaginal cytology to premenopausal values. A dose–response relationship was demonstrated in a study by Henzl and coworkers (1973); postmenopausal women were treated with 5, 20, or 80 mcg of Mestranol per day, and the KPI increased progressively with the dosage.

HRT and Other Menopausal Symptoms

Studies investigating the benefits of HRT on other menopausal symptoms have already been discussed in previous sections of this chapter. With the exception of hot flashes and atrophic vaginitis, the research has not been supportive of HRT as an effective mode of treatment for symptoms commonly attributed to menopause, such as depression, nervousness, insomnia, fatigue, and headaches.

HRT and Hormonal Levels

The assumed mechanism by which HRT acts to improve symptoms of vasomotor instability and atrophic vaginitis is by effecting changes in circulating levels of estrogen and/or gonadotropins. Regardless of the route of administration, HRT administered to postmenopausal women does tend to increase estrone and estradiol concentrations and to reduce FSH and LH. In general, studies have found greater increases in estrone than the more biologically active estradiol (e.g., Lind, 1978) and some reduction in gonadotropins but not to premenopausal levels (e.g., Stumpf et al., 1982). These effects vary with dose and method of administration of HRT; one study (Thom, Collins, & Studd, 1981) found implants to produce extremely elevated levels of estrogen, decreases in FSH to premenopausal values, and less dramatic decreases in LH.

Similar results have been found with acute administration of estrogen. Within several hours after ingestion of 2 mg of micronized estradiol, Yen and colleagues (1975) found significant increases in estradiol and estrone and significant decreases in FSH and LH. Similar results have been reported by Tsai and Yen (1971) and Nillius and Wide (1970). Asch and coworkers (1983) injected oophorectomized rhesus monkeys with estrogen; during the first 24 hours, FSH and LH levels decreased by 70 to 80%, followed by a rebound to 60 to 80% above basal levels at 48 hours. Some animals received additional injections of GnRH, which enhanced the negative feedback of estrogen on gonadotropins and diminished the subsequent positive feedback. The authors interpreted their data to mean that exogenous estrogen influences gonadotropin secretion by its action on hypothalamic GnRH.

Because it is thought that oophorectomy results in a more dramatic decrease in estrogen levels than does natural menopause, oophorectomized women are assumed to be particularly susceptible to symptoms. Thus, HRT is frequently begun immediately following surgery in order to prevent changes in estrogen and gonadotropins. Several studies (Ostergard, Parlow, & Townsend, 1970; Simon & di Zerega, 1982) have noted that, although HRT begun immediately after surgery resulted in a maintenance of presurgical levels of estrogen, LH and FSH increased to typical postmenopausal levels. In contrast, Hunter and colleagues (1977) found that estrogen implants prevented both decreases in estrogen and increases in gonadotropins. However, they did not report the actual levels of circulating estrogen resulting from this procedure, which would be relevant since implants tend to produce levels of estrogen considerably above premenopausal values.

Dose–response relationships between HRT and hormone concentrations have been studied. Mandel and coworkers (1982; 1983) assessed the effects of various doses of exogenous estrogen on estrogen and gonadotropin levels. Stepwise increases in circulating estrone and estradiol occurred with increasing dosages, but none of the doses tested reduced gonadotropins to premenopausal levels. In a similar study, Utian and colleagues (1978) found that the highest dose tested (2.5 mg of conjugated estrogen) reduced FSH, but not LH levels, to premenopausal levels, but it also resulted in estradiol levels higher than those found during premenopause. Assessing four dosages of HRT on a variety of physical and biochemical markers, Geola and coworkers (1980) concluded that determining the optimal dosage was difficult since "All doses exerted subphysiological, physiological, and pharmacological responses at different sites of action" (p. 620).

The most popular form of HRT is oral, but this method is relatively ineffective due to poor gastrointestinal absorption. One method of increasing the effectiveness of oral medication is to provide it in micronized form; micronization increases the surface area by reducing the particle size, thereby facilitating dissolution and absorption. Martin, Burnier, and Greaney (1972) reported that the micronized form was well tolerated and preferred over the regular form by most subjects. However, Casper and Yen (1981) found that, although absorption was extremely rapid, micronized estrogen, like other forms of oral estrogen, resulted in abnormally high elevations of estrone at the dose required to achieve physiological levels of estradiol.

Estrone increases at a faster rate than does estadiol when HRT is administered orally because the intestines and the liver convert estradiol, the more active form of estrogen, to estrone. Other routes of administration have been studied in order to discover a method that might bypass the gut and the liver and avoid the rapid conversion of estradiol to estrone. Several studies have compared oral to cutaneous (usually on the abdomen) administration and have reported that both routes increase estradiol and decrease FSH and LH to similar levels, but that oral administration results in considerably higher levels of estrone than does estrogen applied cutaneously (Elkik et al., 1982; Fahraeus & Larsson-Cohn, 1982; Lyrenas et al., 1981). Fahraeus, Larsson-Cohn, and Wallentin (1982) and Fahraeus and Wallentin (1983) compared these two methods of administration on lipoproteins. Both studies reported a change in lipoproteins with oral but not with cutaneous administration; however, the changes noted with the oral route could be viewed as beneficial ones with respect to atherosclerotic disease.

A second alternative method of administering HRT is intravaginally, which, as does the cutaneous route, bypasses the gut and liver. Deutsch, Ossowski, and Benjamin (1981) compared vaginal to oral administration at a variety of dosages and found that, at each dosage level, the vaginal route resulted in significantly lower blood estrogen values than did the oral route. However, relief from vaginal symptoms was achieved in all cases where the hormone was administered vaginally. Rigg and coworkers (1977) compared vaginal to intranasal administration, and a lower ratio of estrone to estradiol was obtained with the vaginal route. These data are consistent with those comparing oral and cutaneous administrations in that routes of administration that bypass the gut and liver produce a more physiological ratio of estrone to estradiol.

HRT and Cancer

There is considerable evidence that exogenous estrogen treatment in menopausal women is associated with an increase in the probability of developing uterine cancer. Studies comparing the rate of uterine cancer among women receiving estrogen therapy to those not receiving such therapy have estimated the increased risk associated with estrogen to be four to eight times (Gambrell et al., 1980; Greenwald, Caputo, & Wolfgang, 1977; Hammond et al., 1979; Smith et al., 1975). Stronger evidence for a relationship between exogenous estrogen and uterine cancer comes from studies evaluating the effects of dose and duration of estrogen treatment. Several researchers (Ziel & Finkle, 1975, 1976) found duration of estrogen use to be significantly correlated with risk of uterine cancer, while others (Gray, Christopherson, & Hoover, 1977; Rosenwaks et al., 1979; Stavraky et al., 1981) have found both dose and duration to bear a linear relationship to risk. For example, Ziel and Finkle (1975) reported a risk–ratio estimate of 13.9 for seven years or more of estrogen use.

Predisposing factors for uterine cancer include obesity, hypertension, diabetes, and nulliparity (Buchman, Kramer, & Feldman, 1978). Investigations of interacting and/or additive effects of such predisposing factors and estrogen use on uterine cancer have yielded inconsistent results. Buchman, Kramer, and Feldman (1978) found that virtually all of their subjects with uterine cancer had either at least one of the predisposing factors or had had estrogen therapy. Data presented by Judd and coworkers (1982) indicate that the two groups most susceptible to cancer are obese women and slender women on HRT, but these authors noted that such research is difficult to interpret since obese women may be less likely to be on estrogen. Smith and colleagues (1975) concluded from their research that the increased risk of uterine cancer due to exogenous estrogen is less apparent in patients with characteristics that already predispose them.

The relationship between obesity and uterine cancer and HRT and uterine cancer suggest, perhaps, that increased blood estrogen levels contribute to the development of uterine cancer since obese persons exhibit a higher rate of conversion from androgens to estrogen and, thus, have higher blood concentrations of estrogen. Nisker and coworkers (1980) found sex-hormone-binding globulin levels to be significantly lower and free estradiol levels significantly higher in cancer patients than in controls; however, the cancer patients were also more obese. In two studies comparing estrogen levels of women with and without uterine cancer in which subjects were matched for weight, no differences in serum estrogen levels were found (Judd, Lucas, & Yen, 1976; Lucas & Yen, 1979).

There is some evidence to suggest that the mechanism by which exogenous estrogen predisposes one to uterine cancer is via a direct effect on the endometrium. Exogenous estrogen administration has been shown to be consistently associated with endometrial hyperplasia (Callantine et al., 1975; Sturdee et al., 1978; Whitehead et al., 1978). Aycock and Jollie (1979) compared the cellular response of the postmenopausal endometrium to estrogenic stimulation with the cellular activity in endometrial cancer and found close similarities. Natrajan and colleagues (1981) have suggested that unopposed estrogen stimulation increases the concentration of estrogen receptors, resulting in a state of hyperreceptivity to estrogen, the consequence being hyperplasia and, perhaps, cancer.

There has been considerable controversy over the interpretation of this research and differing conclusions as to the nature of the relationship between exogenous estrogen and uterine cancer ranging from ". . . I am convinced that estrogens per se are not a cause of endometrial cancer in the human female" (Kistner, 1976, p. 479) to ". . . the U.S. may be observing the close of an unparalleled epidemic of drug-induced cancer" (Walker & Hershel, 1980, p. 733). Consequently, the responses of researchers, practitioners, and patients to the increasing evidence of a relationship between HRT and uterine cancer have been mixed. One response of physicians has been to minimize the life-threatening nature of uterine cancer by stating that cancers arising due to estrogen therapy are usually diagnosed early and are readily cured (Chu, Schweid, & Weiss, 1982; Kistner, 1976).

A second response has been to develop other forms of HRT that are not associated with an increased risk of cancer. Initially, hormone replacement therapy consisted of estrogen administered on a continual basis. Since the increased risk of uterine cancer was thought to be due to the hyperplasic effects of unopposed estrogen on the endometrium, other forms of medication have been advocated. For example, estrogen is sometimes given on a cyclic basis, with 25 days of medication and 5 days off, in order to prevent continuous stimulation of the endometrium. The more common alternative, however, has been to administer estrogen on a cyclic basis and to add progesterone the last 5 to 10 days of the cycle. The rationales for this form of treatment are that it more precisely conforms to premenopausal hormonal levels and, more importantly, that it prevents hyperplasia. Sturdee and coworkers (1978) noted that cyclical unopposed estrogen was associated with a 12% incidence of endometrial hyperplasia, which was reduced to 8% in women with 5 days of progesterone, and there was no case of hyperplasia among women with 10 to 13 days of progesterone. Similar results were reported by Whitehead and colleagues (1978): high-dose cyclical estrogen resulted in a 32% incidence of hyperplasia and low-dose estrogen in a 16% incidence, while estrogen and progesterone administered sequentially resulted in a 6% incidence of hyperplasia with high doses and 3% with low doses. Several researchers (Lind et al., 1979; Flowers, Wilborn, & Hyde, 1983) in this area, however, warn that adding progesterone does not produce regular endometrial shedding in all women, and it should not be assumed that sequential hormonal therapy entirely eliminates the risk of uterine cancer associated with HRT.

The effect of estrogen on the endometrial lining of the uterus is growth, and continual estrogen causes continual growth with haphazard shedding when the lining outgrows its blood supply. According to Budoff (1980), the mechanism by which progesterone protects against hyperplasia is to cause differentiation, and thus, when progesterone and estrogen levels decline, the lining cleanly and precisely sloughs off. King and coworkers (1978) postulate that estrogen increases receptor production in the uterus for both estrogen and progesterone, and that progesterone reduces the concentration of estrogen receptors so that during progesterone therapy the uterus becomes less responsive to estrogen. Support for these effects have been reported by Natrajan and colleagues (1981) who assessed the concentrations of estrogen and progesterone receptors in endometrial biopsies of women receiving estrogen alone and those receiving estrogen plus progesterone. Women receiving high doses of estrogen with progesterone or moderate doses of estrogen without progesterone exhibited significantly elevated concentrations of estrogen receptors, while those receiving moderate doses of estrogen with progesterone exhibited estrogen and progesterone receptor concentrations similar to premenopausal women's in the proliferative phase of the cycle.

Exogenous estrogen has also been linked to cancer of the breast, although there is less research in this area and the results of the available research are inconsistent. Three studies (Hoover et al., 1976; Hulka et al., 1982; Ross et al., 1980) noted an increased risk of breast cancer with estrogen use, while two studies (Gambrell, Maier, & Sanders, 1983; Nachtigall et al., 1979b) found a decreased risk in those on hormones. In the study by Gambrell, Maier, and Sanders (1983), women receiving exogenous estrogen exhibited less risk of breast cancer than untreated controls, and the addition of progesterone to the therapeutic regimen decreased the risk even further.

HRT and Blood Coagulation

As with estrogen in the form of oral contraceptives, estrogen in the form of HRT has been found to affect blood coagulation adversely by causing a change in the biochemical profile in the direction of increased coagulability (Beller, Nachtigall, & Rosenberg, 1972; Coope, Thomson, & Poller, 1975; Poller, Thomson, & Coope, 1980). Some researchers who have reported similar effects of exogenous estrogen on coagulation parameters have interpreted their data as implying a minimal threat for the development of intravascular clots (Stangel et al., 1977; von Kaulla, Droegemueller, & von Kaulla, 1975). On the other hand, they suggest that, although a hypercoagulable state does not imply the necessary formation of a clot, the effects of such a state may be additive with the effects of other predisposing factors frequent in the elderly, such as vascular endothelial damage or prolonged stasis.

Other research has not supported the increased potential toward coagulation from estrogen. Studd and colleagues (1978) and Notelovitz and coworkers (1983) found no evidence for increased coagulability from exogenous estrogen. Methodological differences, such as choice of dependent measure, type of estrogen, and dose and duration of treatment, are probably the cause of these contradictory results, and there has been no systematic evaluation of the relationship between these procedural variations and coagulation. Hunter, Anderson, and Haddon (1979) found changes in the direction of hypercoagulability in women on HRT but qualified their conclusions by stating that the dose tested was higher than that required to relieve hot flashes, and lower doses may have less effect on coagulation (they do not explain why doses above those required to relieve hot flashes were used). A final consideration on this issue is suggested by the results of a study by Notelovitz and colleagues (1981) in which it was found that natural menopause is associated with a shift away from clot formation and toward clot inhibition; thus, exogenous estrogen may change parameters in the direction of clot formation, but this change may simply be a return to the premenopausal level of coagulability and not reflect an abnormal state. Furthermore, since the liver is assumed to be responsible for these changes in coagulation parameters, these changes may be lessened by administration via vaginal or cutaneous routes.

HRT and Other Side Effects

Since a considerable number of postmenopausal women have taken HRT, there has been a readily available population for the investigation of various side effects associated with the use of such medications. The research concerned with the effects of exogenously administered estrogen on carbohydrate metabolism is discussed elsewhere and indicates that, in general, exogenous estrogen tends to cause an increase in blood glucose levels and progesterone has no effect or causes a decrease in blood glucose levels.

The effects of HRT on cholesterol and triglycerides appear to depend on the hormonal content of the medication. HRT containing only estrogen has been found either to increase cholesterol and triglyceride levels significantly (Molitch, Oill, & Odell, 1974) or not to be associated with significant changes in serum cholesterol or triglyceride levels (Walter & Jensen, 1977). Lack of significant changes with estrogen therapy was also reported by Paterson and coworkers (1980); however, they also tested the effects of other compounds and found sequential estrogen/progesterone preparations to reduce serum cholesterol to a level similar to that found in premenopausal women; the effect of triglycerides was significant, but the direction of the change was dependent upon the exact chemical form of the estrogen and progesterone. In another study by the same authors (Paterson et al., 1979), untreated postmenopausal women had significantly higher levels of serum cholesterol than did premenopausal women, and sequential hormone therapy for two months significantly reduced these levels. Serum triglycerides were not significantly elevated in untreated postmenopausal women, and hormone therapy resulted in a significant increase. Finally, Paterson (1982) noted that HRT containing only progesteronic compounds significantly reduced both serum cholesterol and triglycerides.

All the studies discussed above utilized oral forms of HRT. Since the effects of hormones on cholesterol and triglycerides are probably mediated by the liver, nonoral administration may avoid such effects. Mandel and colleagues (1983) assessed the effects of four doses of conjugated estrogen administered vaginally. Although the higher dosages significantly increased hepatic protein synthesis, no dose had a significant effect on circulating levels of triglycerides or cholesterol levels. On the other hand, the decreased levels of cholesterol found with oral administration of sequential compounds may be considered desirable.

Alternative Treatments

Although most hormonal regimens consist of either estrogen alone or estrogen plus progesterone, progesterone alone has also been evaluated as a form of HRT to reduce menopausal symptoms. Progesterone has been found to reduce the frequency of hot flashes (Morrison et al., 1980) and to reduce levels of FSH and LH (Franchimont et al., 1970) in postmenopausal women. Bullock, Massey, and Gambrell (1975) reported that injectable Depo-Provera, a progesterone compound, resulted in the relief of hot flashes and in atrophic endometria but had no effect on vaginal smears. Dennerstein and colleagues (1978) compared the effectiveness of estrogen, progesterone, and a sequential administration of both and found all hormonal preparations to be more effective at reducing vasomotor symptoms than placebo, but regimens containing estrogen were more effective than those with progesterone alone.

Other treatments for vasomotor symptoms associated with menopause have been evaluated, but to a lesser extent than hormonal therapy. Clonidine, an alpha-receptor agonist, is, in high doses, an antihypertensive agent and has been employed as a prophylaxis of migraine headache because of its assumed ability to diminish vascular reactivity. Clayden and coworkers (1974) and Tulandi and colleagues (1983) have evaluated the effectiveness of clonidine in reducing menopausal hot flashes. Both studies found clonidine to be significantly more effective than placebo. Tulandi and coworkers

(1983) also reported that clonidine, while reducing the subjective perceptions of flashes, had no discernible effect on episodic elevations of skin temperature nor on the number of LH peaks. Laufer and colleagues (1982) compared various doses of clonidine to a placebo and found clonidine to be significantly more effective; however, the highest dose, .4 mg/day, reduced the frequency of hot flashes by only 46%, and four of the ten subjects had to discontinue the medication because of severe side effects.

Coope, Williams, and Patterson (1978) administered propranolol, an adrenergic beta-receptor blocking agent effective in treating palpitation and tachycardia, to menopausal women suffering from hot flashes and reported no significant improvement due to the drug. Finally, because of the temporal proximity of hot flashes and LH pulses, Lightman, Jacobs, and Maguire (1982) attempted to treat hot flashes with a GnRH analogue. Initially LH increased dramatically, and within one week levels fell to pretreatment values and remained within the postmenopausal range. Although levels neither of LH nor of FSH were significantly reduced during the five-week treatment period, the treatment was effective in abolishing the pulsatile release of LH in all subjects. Unfortunately, the frequency of subjectively reported hot flashes remained unaltered. The authors concluded that although the pulsatile release of LH is temporally associated with the occurrence of a hot flash, the relationship is not a causal one.

Summary

Hormone replacement therapy is the most common form of treatment for menopausal symptoms, and the research clearly indicates that this treatment is effective in alleviating vasomotor instability and atrophic vaginitis. On the other hand, as discussed in previous sections of this chapter, there is little empirical evidence to endorse treatment with hormones in order to alleviate psychological symptoms or to treat or prevent osteoporosis. The increased risk of uterine cancer associated with HRT renders this form of treatment less than ideal. Anecdotal evidence from my own research in this area suggests that, perhaps, stress reduction, a regular exercise program, and/or vitamin E therapy are useful in reducing the frequency and severity of hot flashes, although none of these have yet been tested empirically for their effectiveness. As the research on HRT becomes more widely available, physicians will be more reluctant to prescribe it and women more reluctant to take it. Consequently, researchers in both medical and nonmedical areas may be motivated to develop and test alternative forms of treatment.

There is apparent, in most of the literature on HRT, an underlying conceptual framework within which menopause, and not the symptoms associated with menopause, is viewed as the problem to be treated. This attitude is apparent in such statements as

> The menopause constitutes a serious emotional event in the life of a woman, and severe psychic manifestations are frequent. It is now widely recognized that ovarian deficiency is the cause of these manifestations. Understanding, and a realization of this fact by every physician and by every woman is vital. This knowledge will undoubtedly favor an aggressive therapeutic approach to estrogen replacement therapy for most menopausal women on a life-long basis (Jern, 1973, p. xiii).

And

> . . . estrogen insufficiency, whether it occurs prior to puberty, during the childbearing years, or at the menopause, represents an abnormal hormonal state that deserves therapeutic correction (Kistner, 1976, p. 479).

Further evidence for the pervasiveness of this perspective is the greater interest in the effects of HRT on blood estrogen levels than on the alleviation of symptoms. A considerable amount of research has been done on the effects of dosage, chemical configuration, and mode of administration of HRT on plasma concentrations of estrogen, LH, and FSH; resulting concentrations are typically compared to those found in premenopausal women. The underlying, and often explicitly stated, justification for such research is that the purpose of HRT is to restore premenopausal levels of these hormones, particularly of estrogen. Since the severity and frequency of hot flashes are not necessarily related to hormone levels, this rationale implies a belief that menopause, itself, is the disorder to be treated.

The view that menopause is a disease and the goal of HRT is to restore the premenopausal physiological state can, perhaps, be explained within a sociocultural framework. The roles for women in our society have traditionally been the biological ones of having and raising children; thus, the physiological state of their reproductive years is considered normal and ideal, and efforts are made to maintain this state. Biology in men, on the other hand, is viewed as secondary in importance to their abilities to think, to perform, and to earn money; although levels of testosterone in men diminish rapidly after the age of 40, testosterone replacement therapy is not typically recommended. Nevertheless, attributing the disease concept of menopause to cultural values does not negate the fact that two symptoms clearly related to menopausal status—hot flashes and atrophic vaginitis—can be disabling or particularly distressing for some women. HRT does reliably alleviate these symptoms in most women, and, if a woman can avoid the discomfort without exposing herself to an unacceptably high risk of cancer, cyclical estrogen with progesterone added during the last ten days of the cycle is the current treatment of choice. Future research in this area should not only develop and evaluate alternative forms of treatment but should also be concerned with determining the lowest dose of HRT that is effective in alleviating hot flashes and atrophic vaginitis and should investigate the possibility of gradually diminishing the dose of HRT without a recurrence of symptoms.

16

Conclusions

Research concerned with the etiology of menopausal symptoms has been characterized by a strong focus on biomedical conceptualizations and methodologies. As a result of such a focus, the physiological event of menopause has been emphasized, and the sociological and psychological aspects of the climacteric transition have been virtually ignored. Although most symptoms that occur prior to and subsequent to menopause probably have multiple interacting etiologies, the research, in general, indicates that only hot flashes and atrophic vaginitis are best viewed within the context of a biological orientation. Other menopausal symptoms, such as depression, anxiety, fatigue, and weight gain, would, perhaps, be more appropriately termed climacteric symptoms, since the evidence suggests that these symptoms bear a stronger relationship to the stress associated with and the psychological manifestations of cultural attitudes toward aging and menopause than to physiology.

Since the literature concerned with the treatment of menopausal symptoms is also almost exclusively grounded in a biomedical conceptualization system, this body of literature is relevant to only a few of the many difficulties women experience during the climacteric transition. Tranquilizers and individual psychotherapy have occasionally been advocated for those symptoms that do not respond to hormonal treatment. However, such treatment must be viewed as symptomatic rather than curative, since the problem is not one of individual psychopathology but one of cultural pathology. Although cultural values and attitudes are not easily nor readily modified, newly developing areas in sociology, psychology, and medicine are beginning to focus on system-centered rather than person-centered theories, and the eventual application of these theories may provide a context for viewing menopause as a natural, and potentially positive, experience in which freedom and wisdom rather than childbearing and youthful beauty are emphasized and valued.

In conclusion, although menopause strictly refers to a physiological event—the cessation of menses—the psychological manifestations and social impact and implications of menopause cannot be ignored in the study of symptoms associated with menopause. Women's roles have traditionally been limited to biological ones, women's femininity has been judged according to their reproductive capacity, and their value has depended upon their youth and beauty. Thus, although aging is psychologically difficult for everyone to accept, it is not surprising that it is particularly difficult for women, and menopause is clearly a sign of aging. Discussions in previous chapters indicate that stress, beliefs, and attitudes can and do influence central and peripheral nervous system activity, reactivity to stress, susceptibility to disease, psychological and behavioral parameters, and the subjective report of symptoms. Thus, the study of menopause necessitates the consideration of psychological, social, and cultural, as well as physiological, factors.

References

Abe, T., Furuhashi, N., Yamaya, Y., Wada, Y., Hoshiai, A., and Suzuki, M. (1977). Correlation between climacteric symptoms and serum levels of estradiol, progesterone, follicle-stimulating hormone, and lutenizing hormone. *American Journal of Obstetrics and Gynecology, 129*, 65–67.

Abplanalp, J. M., Donnelly, A. F., and Rose, R. M. (1979). Psychoendocrinology of the menstrual cycle: I. Enjoyment of daily activities and mood. *Psychosomatic Medicine, 41*, 587–604.

Abplanalp, J. M., Livingston, L., Rose, R. M., and Sandwisch, D. (1977). Cortisol and growth hormone responses to psychological stress during the menstrual cycle. *Psychosomatic Medicine, 39*, 158–77.

Abplanalp, J. M., Rose, R. M., Donnelly, A. F., and Livingston-Vaughan, L. (1979). Psychoendocrinology of the menstrual cycle: II. The relationship between enjoyment of activities, moods, and reproductive hormones. *Psychosomatic Medicine, 41*, 605–15.

Abramson, M., and Torghele, J. R. (1961). Weight, temperature changes and psychosomatic symptomatology in relation to the menstrual cycle. *American Journal of Obstetrics and Gynecology, 81*, 223–32.

Adamopoulos, D. A., Loraine, J. A., and Dove, G. A. (1971). Endocrinological studies in women approaching the menopause. *Journal of Obstetrics and Gynecology of the British Commonwealth, 78*, 62–79.

Adams, P. W., Rose, D. P., Folkard, J., Wynn, V., Seed, M., and Strong, R. (1973). Effect of pyridoxine hydrochloride (Vitamin B_6) upon depression associated with oral contraception. *Lancet*, April, 897–904.

Aitken, J. M. (1976). Bone metabolism in post-menopausal women. In R. J. Beard (Ed.), *The Menopause: A Guide to Current Research & Practice*. Baltimore, Md.: University Park Press.

Aitken, J. M., Hart, D. M., Anderson, J. B., Lindsay, R., Smith, D. A., and Speirs, C. F. (1973). Osteoporosis after oophorectomy for non-malignant disease in premenopausal women. *British Medical Journal, ii*, 325–28.

Ajabor, L. N., Tsai, C. C., Vela, P., and Yen, S. S. C. (1972). Effect of exogenous estrogen on carbohydrate metabolism in postmenopausal women. *American Journal of Obstetrics and Gynecology, 113,* 383–87.

Akerlund, M., and Andersson, K. E. (1976). Effects of terbutaline on human myometrial activity and endometrial blood flow. *Obstetrics and Gynecology, 47,* 529–35.

Akerlund, M., Andersson, K. E., and Ingemarsson, I. (1976). Effects of terbutaline on myometrial activity, uterine blood flow, and lower abdominal pain in women with primary dysmenorrhea. *British Journal of Obstetrics and Gynecology, 83,* 673–78.

Akerlund, M., Stromberg, P., and Forsling, M. L. (1979). Primary dysmenorrhea and vasopressin. *British Journal of Obstetrics and Gynecology, 86,* 484–87.

Akil, H., Watson, S. J., Young, E., Lewis, M. E., Khactaturian, H., and Walker, J. M. (1984). Endogenous opioids: Biology and function. *Annual Review of Neuroscience, 7,* 223–55.

Akiskal, H. S. (1979). A biochemical approach to depression. In R. A. Depue, *The Psychology of the Depressive Disorders: Implications for the Effects of Stress.* New York: Academic Press.

Aksel, S. (1979). Luteinizing hormone-releasing hormone and the human menstrual cycle. *American Journal of Obstetrics and Gynecology, 135,* 96–101.

____ (1981). On the correlation of luteinizing hormone-releasing hormone, luteinizing hormone, follicle-stimulating hormone, and prolactin levels in plasma of women with normal menstrual cycles. *American Journal of Obstetrics and Gynecology, 141,* 362–67.

Aksel, S., Schomberg, D. W., and Hammond, C. B. (1977). Prostaglandin F_{2a} production by the human ovary. *Obstetrics and Gynecology, 50,* 347–50.

Aksel, S., Schomberg, D. W., Tyrey, L., and Hammond, C. B. (1976). Vasomotor symptoms, serum estrogens and gonadotropin levels in surgical menopause. *American Journal of Obstetrics and Gynecology, 126,* 165–69.

Altmann, M., Knowles, E., and Bull, H. D. (1941). A psychosomatic study of the sex cycle in women. *Psychosomatic Medicine, 3,* 199–225.

Amin, E-S., El-Sayed, M. M., El-Gamel, B., and Nayel, S. A. (1980). Comparative study of the effect of oral contraceptives containing 50 μg of estrogen and those containing 20 μg of estrogen on adrenal cortical function. *American Journal of Obstetrics and Gynecology, 137,* 831–33.

Andersch, B., Hahn, L., Andersson, M., and Isaksson, B. (1978). Body water and weight in patients with premenstrual tension. *British Journal of Obstetrics and Gynecology, 85,* 549–50.

Andersen, A. N., Larsen, J. F., Steenstrup, O. R., Svendstrup, B., and Nielsen, J. (1977). Effect of bromocriptine on the premenstrual syndrome. A double-blind clinical trial. *British Journal of Obstetrics and Gynecology, 84,* 370–74.

Anderson, A. B. M., Haynes, P. J., Guillebaud, J., and Turnbull, A. C. (1976). Reduction of menstrual blood-loss by prostaglandin-synthetase inhibitors. *Lancet,* April, 774–76.

Anderson, S. G., and Hackshaw, B. T. (1974). The effect of estrogen on uterine blood flow and its distribution in nonpregnant ewes. *American Journal of Obstetrics and Gynecology, 119,* 589–95.

Anisman, H. (1978). Neurochemical changes elicited by stress: Behavioral correlates. In H. Anisman and G. Bignami (Eds.), *Psychopharmacology of Aversively Motivated Behavior.* New York: Plenum.

Anton-Tay, F., and Wurtman, R. J. (1968). Norepinephrine: Turnover in rat brains after gonadectomy. *Science, 159,* 1245.

Anzalone, M. K. (1977). Postpartum depression and premenstrual tension, life stress, and marital adjustment. Unpublished doctoral dissertation, Boston University.

Appleby, B. P. (1960). A study of premenstrual tension in general practice. *British Medical Journal,* February, 391–93.

Archer, D. F. (1982). Biochemical findings and medical management of menopause. In A. M. Voda, M. Dinnerstein, and S. R. O'Connell, *Changing Perspectives on Menopause.* Austin: University of Texas Press.

Arrata, W. S. M., and Chatterton, R. T. (1974). Effect of prostaglandin F_{2a} on the luteal phase of the cycle in nonpregnant women. *American Journal of Obstetrics and Gynecology, 120,* 954–59.

Arrata, W. S. M., and Tsai, A. Y. M. (1978). Prostaglandins in reproduction. *Journal of Reproductive Medicine, 20,* 84–88.

Asch, E. H., Balmaceda, J. P., Borghi, M. R., Niesvisky, R., Coy, D. H., and Schally, A. V. (1983). Suppression of the positive feedback of estradiol benzoate on gonadotropin secretion by an inhibitory analog of luteinizing hormone-releasing hormone (LRH) in oophorectomized rhesus monkeys: Evidence for a necessary synergism between LRH and estrogens. *Journal of Clinical Endocrinology & Metabolism, 57,* 367–72.

Aslan, S., Nelson, L., Carruthers, M., and Lader, M. (1981). Stress and age effects on catecholamines in normal subjects. *Journal of Psychosomatic Research, 25,* 33–41.

Averill, J. R. (1979). A selective review of cognitive and behavioral factors involved in the regulation of stress. In R. A. Depue, *The Psychology of the Depressive Disorders: Implications for the Effects of Stress.* New York: Academic Press.

Aycock, N. R., and Jollie, W. P. (1979). Ultrastructural effects of estrogen replacement on postmenopausal endometrium. *American Journal of Obstetrics and Gynecology, 135,* 461–66.

Backstrom, C. T., Boyle, H., and Baird, D. T. (1981). Persistence of symptoms of premenstrual tension in hysterectomized women. *British Journal of Obstetrics and Gynecology, 88,* 530–36.

Backstrom, T., and Mattsson, B. (1975). Correlation of symptoms in premenstrual tension to oestrogen and progesterone concentrations in blood plasma. *Neuropsychobiology, 1,* 89–86.

Backstrum, R., and Aakvaag, A. (1981). Plasma prolactin and testosterone during the luteal phase in women with premenstrual tension syndrome. *Psychoneuroendocrinology, 6,* 245–51.

Badano, A. R., Nagle, C. A., Casas, P. R. F., Miechi, H., Mirkin, A., Turner, D. E., Aparicio, N., and Rosner, J. M. (1978). Plasma levels of norepinephrine during the periovulatory period in normal women. *American Journal of Obstetrics and Gynecology, 131,* 299–303.

Badawy, S. Z. Z., Elliott, L. J., Elbadawi, A., and Marshall, L. D. (1979). Plasma levels of oestrone and oestradiol-17B in postmenopausal women. *British Journal of Obstetrics and Gynecology, 86,* 56–63.

Baker, A. H., Mishara, B. L., Kostin, I. W., and Parker, L. (1979). Menstrual cycle affects kinesthetic aftereffect, an index of personality and perceptual style. *Journal of Personality and Social Psychology, 37,* 234–46.

Ballinger, C. B. (1975). Psychiatric morbidity and the menopause: Screening of general population sample. *British Medical Journal*, 3, 344–46.

___ (1976). Subjective sleep disturbance at menopause. *Journal of Psychosomatic Research*, *20*, 509–13.

Baran, D. T., Whyte, M. P., Haussler, M. R., Deftos, L. J., Slatopolsky, E., and Avioli, L. V. (1980). Effect of the menstrual cycle on calcium-regulating hormones in the normal young woman. *Journal of Clinical Endocrinology and Metabolism*, *50*, 377–79.

Barnes, R. F., Raskind, M., Gumbrecht, G., and Halter, J. B. (1982). The effects of age on the plasma catecholamine reponse to mental stress in man. *Journal of Clinical Endocrinology and Metabolism*, *54*, 64–69.

Bart, P. B. (1969). Why women's status changes in middle age: The turns of the social ferris wheel. *Sociological Symposium*, Fall, 1–14.

___ (1971). Depression in middle-aged women. In V. Gornick and B. K. Moran (Eds.), *Woman in Sexist Society: Studies in Power and Powerless*. New York: New American Library.

Bart, P. B., and Grossman, M. (1978). Menopause. In M. T. Notman and C. C. Nadelson (Eds.), *Sexual & Reproductive Aspects of Women's Health Care*. New York: Plenum.

Bart, P., and Perlmutter, E. (1981). The menopause in changing times. In B. Justice and R. Pore (Eds.), *Toward the Second Decade: The Impact of the Women's Movement on American Institutions*. Westport, Conn.: Greenwood.

Batta, S. K., Zanisi, M., and Martini, L. (1975). Role of prostaglandins in the control of gonadotropin secretion. *Psychopharmacology*, *1*, 115–21.

Baumblatt, M. J., and Winston, F. (1970). Pyridoxine and the pill. *Lancet*, April, 832.

Baumgardner, S. B., Condrea, H., Daane, T. A., Dorsey, J. H., Jurow, H. N., Shively, J. P., Wachsman, M., Wharton, L. R., and Zibel, M. J. (1978). Replacement estrogen therapy for menopausal vasomotor flushes: Comparison of Quinestrol and conjugated estrogens. *Obstetrics and Gynecology*, *51*, 445–52.

Beard, R. W., Belsey, E. M., Leiberman, B. A., and Wilkinson, J. C. M. (1977). Pelvic pain in women. *American Journal of Obstetrics and Gynecology*, *128*, 566–70.

Beardwood, C. J., Mundrell, C. A., and Utian, W. H. (1975). Gonadotropin excretion in response to audiostimulation of human subjects. American Journal of Obstetrics and Gynecology, 121, 682–87.

Beaumont, P. J. V., Richards, D. H., and Gelder, M. G. (1975). A study of minor psychiatric and physical symptoms during the menstrual cycle. British Journal of Psychiatry, 126, 431–34.

Beck, R. P., Morcos, F., Fawcett, D., and Watanabe, M. (1972). Adrenocortical function studies during the normal menstrual cycle and in women receiving norethindrone with and without mestranol. American Journal of Obstetrics and Gynecology, 112, 364–68.

Beller, F. K., Nachtigall, L., and Rosenberg, M. (1972). Coagulation studies of menopausal women taking estrogen replacement. Obstetrics and Gynecology, 39, 775–78.

Belmaker, R. H., Murphy, D. L., Wyatt, R. J., and Loriaux, D. L. (1974). Human platelet monoamine oxidase changes during the menstrual cycle. Archives of General Psychiatry, 31, 553–56.

Benedek-Jaszmann, L. J., and Hearn-Sturtevant, M. D. (1976). Premenstrual tension and functional infertility. Lancet, May, 1095–98.

Bercovici, B., Uretzki, G., and Patti, Y. (1972). The effects of estrogens on cytology and vascularization of the vaginal epithelium in climacteric women. American Journal of Obstetrics and Gynecology, 113, 98–103.

Bernstein, B. E. (1977). Effect of menstruation on academic performance among college women. Archives of Sexual Behavior, 6, 289–96.

Berry, C., and McQuire, F. L. (1972). Menstrual distress and acceptance of sexual role. American Journal of Obstetrics and Gynecology, 114, 83–87.

Bertoli, A., de Pirro, R., Fusco, A., Greco, A. V., Magnatta, R., and Lauro, R. (1980). Differences in insulin receptors between men and menstruating women and influence of sex hormones on insulin binding during menstrual cycle. Journal of Clinical Endocrinology and Metabolism, 50, 246–50.

Bickers, W. B. (1954). Menorrhalgia—Menstrual Distress. Springfield, Ill.: Charles C Thomas.

—— (1941). Uterine contractions in dysmenorrhea. American Journal of Obstetrics and Gynecology, 42, 1023–30.

Birtchnell, J., and Floyd, S. (1975). Attempted suicide and the menstrual cycle—A negative conclusion. *Journal of Psychosomatic Research, 8,* 361–69.

Bloom, L. J., Shelton, J. L., and Michaels, A. C. (1978). Dysmenorrhea and personality. *Journal of Personality Assessment, 42,* 272–76.

Bolognese, R. J., and Corson, S. L. (1973). The effect of vaginally administered prostaglandin F_{2a} on corpus luteum function. *American Journal of Obstetrics and Gynecology, 117,* 240–45.

Bolton, R. A., Coulam, C. B., and Ryan, R. J. (1980). Specific binding of human chorionic gonadotropin to human corpora lutea in the menstrual cycle. *Obstetrics and Gynecology, 56,* 336–38.

Bottari, S. P., Bokaer, A., Kaivez, E., Lescrainier, P., and Vauquelin, G. P. (1983). Differential regulation of a-adrenergic receptor subclasses by gonadal steroids in human myometrium. *Journal of Clinical Endocrinology and Metabolism, 57,* 937–41.

Brehm, J. W. (1966). *A Theory of Psychological Reactance.* New York: Academic Press.

Brockway, J. (1975). Prediction of premenstrual symptomatology using the Moos Menstrual Distress Questionnaire. Unpublished doctoral dissertation, University of Iowa.

Brooks-Gunn, J., and Ruble, D. (1979). Dysmenorrhea in adolescence. Paper presented at the APA, New York, September.

—— (1980a). Menarche: The interaction of physiological, cultural, and social factors. In A. J. Dan, E. A. Graham, and C. P. Beecher (Eds.), *The Menstrual Cycle: Volume 1: A Synthesis of Interdisciplinary Research.* New York: Springer Publishing.

—— (1980b). The menstrual attitude questionnaire. *Psychosomatic Medicine, 42,* 503–12.

Brown, J. J., Davies, D. L., Lever, A. F., and Robertson, J. I. S. (1964). Variations in plasma renin during the menstrual cycle. *British Medical Journal,* October, 1114–15.

Buchman, M. I., Kramer, E., and Feldman, G. B. (1978). Aspiration curettage for asymptomatic patients receiving estrogen. *Obstetrics and Gynecology, 51,* 339–41.

Buckman, M. T., Peake, G. T., and Srivastava, L. S. (1976). Endogenous estrogen modulates phenothiazine stimulated prolactin secretion. *Journal of Clinical Endocrinology and Metabolism, 43,* 901-6.

Buckman, M. T., and Peake, G. T. (1973). Estrogen potentiation of phenothiazine-induced prolactin secretion in man. *Journal of Clinical Endocrinology and Metabolism, 37,* 977–80.

Budoff, P. W. (1980). *No More Menstrual Cramps and Other Good News.* New York: G. P. Putnam's Sons.

Bullamore, J. R., Gallagher, J. C., Wilkinson, R., Nordin, B. E. C., and Marshall, D. H. (1970). Effect of age on calcium absorption. *Lancet,* September, 535–37.

Bullock, J. L., Massey, F. M., and Gambrell, R. D. (1975). Use of medroxy-progesterone acetate to prevent menopausal symptoms. *Obstetrics and Gynecology, 46,* 165–68.

Burchfield, S. R. (1979). The stress response: A new perspective. *Psychosomatic Medicine, 41,* 661–72.

Burnier, A. M., Martin, P. L., Yen, S. S. C., and Brooks, P. (1981). Sublingual absorption of micronized 17B-estradiol. *American Journal of Obstetrics and Gynecology, 140,* 146–49.

Callantine, M. R., Martin, P. L., Bolding, O. T., Warner, P. O., and Greaney, M. O. (1975). Micronized 17B-estradiol for oral estrogen therapy in menopausal women. *Obstetrics and Gynecology, 46,* 37–41.

Campos, F., and Thurow, C. (1978). Attributions of moods and symptoms to the menstrual cycle. *Personality and Social Psychology Bulletin, 4,* 272–76.

Cane, E. M., and Villee, C. A. (1975). The synthesis of prostaglandin F by human endometrium in organ culture. *Prostaglandins, 1,* 281–87.

Canniggia, A., Gennari, C., Borrello, G., Bencini, M., Cesari, L., Poggi, C., and Escobar, S. (1970). Intestinal absorption of calcium-47 after treatment with oral oestrogen-gestogens in senile osteoporosis. *British Medical Journal, iv,* 30–32.

Carr, B. R., Parker, C. R., Madden, J. D., MacDonald, P. D., and Porter, J. C. (1979). Plasma levels of adrenocorticotropin and cortisol in women receiving oral contraceptive steroid treatment. *Journal of Clinical Endocrinology and Metabolism, 49,* 346–49.

Casper, R. F., and Yen, S. S. C. (1981). Rapid absorption of micronized estradiol-17B following sublingual administration. *Obstetrics and Gynecology, 57,* 62–64.

Casper, R. F., Yen, S. S. C., and Wilkes, M. M. (1979). Menopausal flushes: A neuroendocrine link with pulsatile luteinizing hormone secretion. *Science, 205,* 823–25.

Chakravarti, S., Collins, W. P., Newton, J. R., Oram, D. H., and Studd, J. W. W. (1977). Endocrine changes and symptomatology after oophorectomy in premenopausal women. *British Journal of Obstetrics and Gynecology, 84,* 769–75.

Chan, W. Y., Dawood, M. Y., and Fuchs, F. (1979). Relief of dysmenorrhea with the prostraglandin synthetase inhibitor ibuprofen: Effect on prostaglandin levels in menstrual fluid. *American Journal of Obstetrics and Gynecology, 135,* 102–8.

Chan, W. Y., Fuchs, F., and Powell, A. M. (1983). Effects of naproxen sodium on menstrual prostaglandins and primary dysmenorrhea. *Obstetrics and Gynecology, 61,* 285–91.

Chang, R. J., and Judd, H. L. (1981). The ovary after menopause. *Clinical Obstetrics and Gynecology, 24,* 181–91.

Check, J. H. (1978). Emotional aspects of menstrual dysfunction. *Psychosomatics, 19,* 178–84.

Chernovetz, M. E., Jones, W. H., and Hansson, R. D. (1979). Predictability, attentional focus, sex role orientation, and menstrual-related stress in women. *Psychosomatic Medicine, 41,* 383–91.

Chesney, M. A., and Tasto, D. L. (1975a). The development of the menstrual symptom questionnaire. *Behavior Research and Therapy, 13,* 237–44.

—— (1975b). The effectiveness of behavior modification with spasmodic and congestive dysmenorrhea. *Behavior Research and Therapy, 13,* 245–53.

Christiansen, C., Christensen, M. S., Larsen, N. E., and Transbol, I. (1982). Pathophysiological mechanisms of estrogen effect on bone metabolism. Dose–response relationships in early postmenopausal women. *Journal of Clinical Endocrinology and Metabolism, 55,* 1124–30.

Christie Brown J. R. S., and Christie Brown, M. E. (1976). Psychiatric disorders associated with the menopause. In R. J. Beard (Ed.), *The*

Menopause: A Guide to Current Research & Practice. Baltimore: University Park Press.

Chu, J., Schweid, A. I., and Weiss, N. S. (1982). Survival among women with endometrial cancer: A comparison of estrogen users and non-users. *American Journal of Obstetrics and Gynecology, 143,* 569.

Cibils, L. A. (1971). Effect of mesuprine hydrochloride upon nonpregnant uterine contractility and the cardiovascular system. *American Journal of Obstetrics and Gynecology, 111,* 187–96.

Clark, K. E., Farley, D. B., Van Orden, D. E., and Brody, M. J. (1977). Role of endrogenous prostaglandins in regulation of uterine blood flow and adrenergic transmission. *American Journal of Obstetrics and Gynecology, 127,* 455–61.

Clayden, J. R., Bell, J. W., and Pollard, P. (1974). Menopausal flushing: Double-blind trial of non-hormonal medication. *British Medical Journal, 1,* 409–12.

Cobo, E., Cifuentes, R., and de Villamizar, M. (1978). Inhibition of menstrual uterine motility during water diuresis. *American Journal of Obstetrics and Gynecology, 132,* 313–20.

Cooke, D. J., and Greene, J. G. (1981). Types of life events in relation to symptoms at the climacterium. *Journal of Psychosomatic Research, 25,* 5–11.

Coope, J., Thomson, J. M., and Poller, L. (1975). Effects of "natural oestrogen" replacement therapy on menopausal symptoms and blood clotting. *British Medical Journal,* October, 139–43.

Coope, J., Williams, S., and Patterson, J. S. (1978). A study of the effectiveness of propranolol in menopausal hot flushes. *British Journal of Obstetrics and Gynecology, 85,* 474–75.

Cooper, J. R., Bloom, F. E., and Roth, R. H. (1982). *The Biochemical Basis of Neuropharmacology* (4th ed.). New York: Oxford Press.

Coppen, A., and Kessel, N. (1963). Menstruation and personality. *British Journal of Psychiatry, 109,* 711–21.

Coudert, S. P., Winter, J. S. D., and Faiman, C. (1974). Transient decline in serum progesterone levels during prostaglandin F_{2a} infusion in the midluteal phase of the normal menstrual cycle. *American Journal of Obstetrics and Gynecology, 119,* 755–61.

Coulam, C. B. (1981). Age, estrogen and the psyche. *Clinical Obstetrics and Gynecology, 24,* 219–29.

Coutinho, E. M., and Darze, E. (1976). Spontaneous contractility and the response of the human uterine cervix to prostaglandins F_{2a} and E_2 during the menstrual cycle. *American Journal of Obstetrics and Gynecology, 126,* 224–25.

Coutinho, E. M., and Lopes, A. C. V. (1968). Response of the nonpregnant uterus to vasopressin as an index of ovarian function. *American Journal of Obstetrics and Gynecology, 102,* 479–89.

Cox, D. J. (1977). Menstrual symptom questionnaire: Further psychometric evaluation. *Behavior Research and Therapy, 15,* 506–8.

Cox, D. J., and Meyer, R. G. (1978). Behavioral treatment parameters with primary dysmenorrhea. *Journal of Behavioral Medicine, 1,* 297–310.

Csapo, A. I., and Csapo, E. E. (1974). The "prostaglandin step," a bottleneck in the activation of the uterus. *Life Science, 14,* 719–24.

Csapo, A. I., Pitkanen, Y., and Pulkkinen, M. (1975). The effects of isoxsuprine on uterine contractility. *Obstetrics and Gynecology, 46,* 58–63.

Csapo, A. I., Pulkkinen, M. O., and Henzl, M. R. (1977). The effect of Naproxen-sodium on the intrauterine pressure and menstrual pain of dysmenorrheic patients. *Prostaglandins, 13,* 193–99.

Cudworth, A. G., and Veevers, A. (1975). Carbohydrate metabolism in the menstrual cycle. *British Journal of Obstetrics and Gynecology, 82,* 162–69.

Cullberg, J. (1972). Mood changes and menstrual symptoms with different gestation/estrogen combinations. *Acta Psychiatrica Scandinavica,* Suppl. 236.

Cumming, D. C., Rebar, R. W., Hopper, B. R., and Yen, S. S. C. (1982). Evidence for an influence of the ovary on circulating dehydroepiandrosterone sulfate levels. *Journal of Clinical Endocrinology and Metabolism, 54,* 1069–71.

Cutler, W. B., and Garcia, C. R. (1980). The psychoneuroendocrinology of the ovulatory cycle of women: A review. *Psychoneuroendocrinology, 5,* 89–111.

Czekanowski, R. (1975). Influence of prostaglandins F_{2a} and #1 on vaginal contractility. *Obstetrics and Gynecology, 45,* 628–31.

Dalton, K. (1959a). Comparative trials of new oral progestogenic compounds in treatment of premenstrual syndrome. *British Medical Journal*, December, 1307–9.

___ (1959b). Menstruation and acute psychiatric illness. *British Medical Journal*, January, 148–49.

___ (1960a). Effect of menstruation on school girls' weekly work. *British Medical Journal*, January, 326–28.

___ (1960b). Menstruation and accidents. *British Medical Journal*, November, 1425–26.

___ (1960c). School girls' behavior and menstruation. *British Medical Journal*, December, 1647–49.

___ (1961). Menstruation and crime. *British Medical Journal*, December, 1752–53.

___ (1964). *The Premenstrual Syndrome*. Springfield, Ill.: Charles C Thomas.

___ (1968). Menstruation and examinations. *Lancet*, December, 1386–88.

___ (1980). Cyclical criminal acts in premenstrual syndrome. *Lancet*, ii, 1070–71.

Dan, A. J., Graham, E. A., Beecher, C. P., Bart, P. B., Komenish, P., Krueger, J., Pitel, M., and Ruble, D. Synthesis and new directions. In A. J. Dan, E. A. Graham, and C. P. Beecher (Eds.), *The Menstrual Cycle, Volume 1: A Synthesis of Interdisciplinary Research*. New York: Springer Publishing.

Davidson, B. J., Riggs, B. L., Wahner, H. W., and Judd, H. L. (1983). Endogenous cortisol and sex steroids in patients with osteoporotic spinal fractures. *Obstetrics and Gynecology, 61*, 275–78.

Davidson, B. J., Ross, R. K., Paganini-Hill, A., Hammond, G., Siiteri, P. K., and Judd, H. L. (1982). Total and free estrogens and androgens in postmenopausal women with hip fractures. *Journal of Clinical Endocrinology and Metabolism, 54*, 115–20.

Davies, M., Mawer, E. B., and Adams, P. H. (1977). Vitamin D metabolism and the response to 1,25-Dihydroxycholecalciferol in osteoporosis. *Journal of Clinical Endocrinology and Metabolism, 45*, 199–208.

Delaney, J., Lupton, M. J., and Toth, E. (1977). *The Curse: A Cultural History of Menstruation,* New York: New American Library.

Dennerstein, L., Burrows, G. D., Hyman, G., and Wood, C. (1978). Menopausal hot flushes: A double blind comparison of placebo, ethinyl oestradiol and norgestrel. *British Journal of Obstetrics and Gynecology, 85,* 852–56.

Dennerstein, L., Spencer-Gardner, C., Gotts, G., Brown, J., Smith, M., and Burrows, G. (1983). The menstrual cycle—correlating biological and psychological changes. In L. Dennerstein and M. Senarclens (Eds.), *The Young Woman: Psychosomatic Aspects of Obstetrics and Gynecology.* Amsterdam: Excerpta Medica.

de Pirro, R., Fusco, A., Bertoli, A., Greco, A. V., and Lauro, R. (1978). Insulin receptors during the menstrual cycle in normal women. *Journal of Clinical Endocrinology and Metabolism, 47,* 1387–89.

Dege, K., and Gretzinger, J. (1982). Attitudes of families toward menopause. In A. M. Voda, M. Dinnerstein, and S. R. O'Donnell (Eds.), *Changing Perspectives on Menopause.* Austin: University of Texas Press.

Deutsch, S., Ossowski, R., and Benjamin, I. (1981). Comparison between degree of systemic absorption of vaginally and orally administered estrogens at different dose levels in postmenopausal women. *American Journal of Obstetrics and Gynecology, 139,* 967–68.

Dewhurst, C. J. (1976). The role of estrogen in preventative medicine. In R. J. Beard (Ed.), *The Menopause: A Guide to Current Research and Practice.* Baltimore, Md.: University Park Press.

Dimsdale, J. E., and Moss. J. (1980). Short-term catecholamine response to psychological stress. *Psychosomatic Medicine, 42,* 493–97.

DiPaola, G., Robin, M., and Nicholson, R. (1970). Estrogen therapy and glucose tolerance test. *American Journal of Obstetrics and Gynecology, 107,* 124–32.

DiZerega, P. S., Goebelsmann, U., and Nakamura, R. M. (1982). Identification of protein(s) secreted by the preovulatory ovary which suppresses the follicle response to gonadotropins. *Journal of Clinical Endocrinology and Metabolism, 54,* 1091–96.

Donovan, J. C. (1951). The menopausal syndrome: A study of case histories. *American Journal of Obstetrics and Gynecology, 62,* 1281–91.

d'Orban, P. T., and Dalton, K. (1980). Violent crime and the menstrual cycle. *Psychological Medicine, 10,* 353–59.

Dor-Shav, N. K. (1976). In search of pre-menstrual tension: Note on sex differences in psychological differentiation as a function of cyclical physiological changes. *Perceptual and Motor Skills, 42,* 1139–42.

Doty, R. L., Snyder, P. J., Huggins, G. R., and Lowry, L. D. (1981). Endocrine, cardiovascular, and psychological correlates of olfactory sensitivity changes during the human menstrual cycle. *Journal of Comparative and Physiological Psychology, 95,* 45–60.

Downie, S., Poyser, N. L., and Wunderlich, M. (1974). Levels of prostaglandin in human endometrium during the normal menstrual cycle. *Journal of Physiology, 236,* 465–72.

Drake, T. S., O'Brien, W. F., Ramwell, P. W., and Metz, S. A. (1981). Peritoneal fluid thromboxane B_2 and 6-keto-prostaglandin F_{1a} in endometriosis. *American Journal of Obstetrics and Gynecology, 140,* 401–4.

Dyer, D. C., and Gough, E. D. (1971). Comparative actions of selected vasoactive drugs on isolated human uterine arteries. *American Journal of Obstetrics and Gynecology, 111,* 820–25.

Ehara, Y., Siler, T., Vanderberg, G., Sinha, Y. N., and Yen, S. S. C. (1973). Circulating prolactin levels during the menstrual cycle: Episodic release and diurnal variation. *American Journal of Obstetrics and Gynecology, 117,* 962–70.

Ehrenreich, B., and English, D. (1973). *Complaints and Disorders: The Sexual Politics of Sickness.* New York: The Feminist Press.

Elder, M. G., and Kapadia, L. (1979). Indomethacin in the treatment of primary dysmenorrhea. *British Journal of Obstetrics and Gynecology, 86,* 645–47.

Elkik, F., Gompel, A., Mercier-Bodard, C., Kuttenn, F., Guyenne, P. N., Corvol, P., and Mauvais-Jarvis, P. (1982). Effects of percutaneous estradiol and conjugated estrogens on the level of plasma proteins and triglycerides in postmenopausal women. *American Journal of Obstetrics and Gynecology, 143,* 888-92.

Elsner, C. W., Buster, J. E., Schindler, R. A., Nessim, S. A., and Abraham, G. E. (1980). Bromodriptine in the treatment of premenstrual tension syndrome. *Obstetrics and Gynecology, 56,* 723–26.

Engel, B. T. (1960). Stimulus–response and individual-response specificity. *Archives of General Psychiatry, 2,* 305–13.

Englander-Golden, P., Willis, K. A., and Dienstbier, R. A. (1977). Stability of perceived tension as a function of the menstrual cycle. *Journal of Human Stress, 3,* 14–21.

Epstein, M. T., Hockaday, J. M., and Hockaday, T. D. R. (1975). Migraine and reproductive hormones throughout the menstrual cycle. *Lancet,* March, 543–47.

Erlik, Y., Meldrum, D. R., and Judd, H. L. (1982). Estrogen levels in postmenopausal women with hot flashes. *Obstetrics and Gynecology, 59,* 403–7.

Fahraeus, L., and Larsson-Cohn, U. (1982). Oestrogens, gonadotrophins and SHBG during oral and cutaneous administration of oestradiol-17B to menopausal women. *Acta Endocrinologica, 101,* 592–96.

Fahraeus, L., Larsson-Cohn, U., and Wallentin, L. (1982). Lipoproteins during oral and cutaneous administration of oestradiol-l17B to menopausal women. *Acta Endocrinologica, 101,* 597–602.

Fahraeus, L., and Wallentin, L. (1983). High density lipoprotein subfractions during oral and cutaneous administration of 17B-estradiol to menopausal women. *Journal of Clinical Endocrinology and Metabolism, 56,* 797–801.

Feldmann, J., and Brown, G. M. (1976). Endocrine responses to electric shock and avoidance conditioning in the rhesus monkey: Cortisol and growth hormone. *Psychoneuroendocrinology, 1,* 231–42.

Fern, M., Rose, D. P., and Fern, E. B. (1978). Effect of oral contraceptives on plasma androgenic steroids and their precursors. *Obstetrics and Gynecology, 51,* 541–44.

Fessler, L. (1950). The psychopathology of climacteric depression. *Psychoanalytic Quarterly, 19,* 27–41.

Filler, W. W., and Hall, W. C. (1970). Dysmenorrhea and its therapy: A uterine contractility study. *American Journal of Obstetrics and Gynecology, 106,* 104–9.

Flint, M. (1975). The menopause: Reward or punishment? *Psychosomatics, 16,* 161–63.

Flowers, C. E., Wilborn, W. H., and Hyde, B. M. (1983). Mechanisms of uterine bleeding in postmenopausal patients receiving estrogen alone or with a progestin. *Obstetrics and Gynecology, 61,* 135–43.

Fournier, P. J. R., Desjardins, P. D., and Friesen, H. G. (1974). Current understanding of human prolactin physiology and its diagnostic and therapeutic applications: A review. *American Journal of Obstetrics and Gynecology, 118,* 337–43.

Franchimont, P., Dession, G., Ayalon, D., Mutsers, A., and Legros, J. J. (1970). Suppressive action of norethisterone ethanate and acetate on gonadotropin (FSH and LH) levels. *Obstetrics and Gynecology, 36,* 93–100.

Frankenhaeuser, M. (1976). The role of peripheral catecholamines in adaptation to understimulation and overstimulation. In G. Serban (Ed.), *Psychopathology of Human Adaptation.* New York: Plenum.

Frankenhaeuser, M., von Wright, M. R., Collins, A., von Wright, J., Sedvall, G., and Swahn, C. G. (1978). Sex differences in psychoneuroendocrine reactions to examination stress. *Psychosomatic Medicine, 40,* 334–43.

Frey, K. A. (1982). Middle-aged women's experience and perception of menopause. *Women and Health, 6,* 25–36.

Friederich, M. A. (1982). Aging, menopause, and estrogens: The clinician's dilemma. In A. M. Voda, M. Dinnerstein, and S. R. O'Connell (Eds.), *Changing Perspectives on Menopause.* Austin: University of Texas Press.

Frisch, R. E., Canick, J. A., and Tulchinsky, D. (1980). Human fatty marrow aromatizes androgen to estrogen. *Journal of Clinical Endocrinology and Metabolism, 51,* 394–96.

Fritz, M. A., and Speroff, L. (1982). The endocrinology of the menstrual cycle: The interaction of folliculogenesis and neuroendocrine mechanisms. *Fertility and Sterility, 38,* 509–29.

—— (1983). Current concepts of the endocrine characteristics of normal menstrual function: The key to diagnosis and management of menstrual disorders. *Clinical Obstetrics and Gynecology, 26,* 649–89.

Frumar, A. M., Meldrum, D. R., Geola, F., Shamonki, I. M., Tataryn, I. V., Deftos, L. J., and Judd, H. L. (1980). Relationship of fasting urinary calcium to circulating estrogen and body weight in postmenopausal women. *Journal of Clinical Endocrinology and Metabolism, 50,* 70–75.

Fuchs, A. R. (1974). Myometrial response to prostaglandins enhanced by progesterone. *American Journal of Obstetrics and Gynecology, 118,* 1093–98.

—— (1977). Prostaglandins. In F. Fuchs and A. Klopper (Eds.), *Endocrinology of Pregnancy* (2nd ed.). New York: Harper & Row.

Fuchs, A. R., Coutinho, E. J., Xavier, R., Bates, P. E., and Fuchs, F. (1968). Effect of ethanol on the activity of the nonpregnant human uterus and its reactivity to neurohypophyseal hormones. *American Journal of Obstetrics and Gynecology, 101,* 997–1000.

Fuchs, A. R., and Fuchs, F. (1973). Possible mechanisms of the inhibition of labor by ethanol. In J. B. Josimovich (Ed.), *Uterine Contraction— Side Effects of Steroidal Contraceptives.* New York: Wiley.

Fuchs, F., Fuchs, A. T., Poblete, F. F., and Risk, A. (1967). Effect of alcohol on threatened premature labor. *American Journal of Obstetrics and Gynecology, 99,* 627–37.

Gallagher, J. C., and Nordin, B. E. C. (1974). Calcium metabolism and the menopause. In A. S. Curry and J. V. Hewitt (Eds.), *Biochemistry of Women: Clinical Concepts.* Cleveland, Ohio: CRC Press.

Gallagher, J. C., Riggs, B. L., and De Luca, H. F. (1980). Effect of estrogen on calcium absorption and serum vitamin D metabolites in postmenopausal osteoporosis. *Journal of Clinical Endocrinology and Metabolism, 51,* 1359–64.

Gambrell, R. D., Maier, R. C., and Sanders, B. I. (1983). Decreased incidence of breast cancer in postmenopausal estrogen–progestogen users. *Obstetrics and Gynecology, 62,* 435.

Gambrell, R. D., Massey, F. M., Castaneda, T. A., Ugenas, A. J., Ricci, C. A., and Wright, J. M. (1980). Use of progestogen challenge test to reduce the risk of endometrial cancer. *Obstetrics and Gynecology, 55,* 732–38.

Gannon, L., Heiser, P., and Knight, S. (in press). Learned helplessness versus reactance: The effects of sex-role stereotypy. *Sex Roles.*

Garrioch, D. B. (1978). The effect of indomethacin on spontaneous activity in the isolated human myometrium and on the response to oxytocin and prostaglandin. *British Journal of Obstetrics and Gynecology, 85,* 47–52.

Genazzani, A. R., Lemarchand-Beraud, T., Aubert, M. L., and Felber, J. P. (1975). Pattern of plasma ACTH, hGH, and cortisol during the menstrual cycle. *Journal of Clinical Endocrinology and Metabolism, 41,* 431–37.

Geola, F. L., Frumar, A. M., Tataryn, I. V., Lu, K. H., Hershman, J. M., Eggena, P., Sambhi, M. P., and Judd, H. L. (1980). Biological effects of various doses of conjugated equine estrogens in postmenopausal women. *Journal of Clinical Endocrinology and Metabolism, 51,* 620–25.

George, G. C. W., Utian, W. H., Beumont, P. J. V., and Beardwood, C. J. (1973). Effect of exogenous oestrogens on minor psychiatric symptoms in postmenopausal women. *South African Medical Journal, 47,* 2387–88.

Gerdes, L. C., EtPhil, D. L., Sonnendecker, E. W. W., and Polakow, E. S. (1982). Psychological changes effected by estrogen-progesterone and clonidine treatment in climacteric women. *American Journal of Obstetrics and Gynecology, 142,* 98–104.

Gerrard, M., Denney, D. R., and Basgall, J. (1979). Pain management and imagery training in the reduction of dysmenorrhea. Paper presented at the American Psychological Association Meeting, New York.

Ghose, K., and Coppen, A. (1977). Bromocriptine and premenstrual syndrome: A controlled study. *British Medical Journal,* January, 147–48.

Gibor, Y., Pandya, G. N., Bieniarz, J., and Scommegna, A. (1971). Uterine contractility and plasma progesterone levels in the nonpregnant woman. *American Journal of Obstetrics and Gynecology, 109,* 542–47.

Gilmore, N. J., Robinson, D. S., Nies, A., Sylwester, D., and Ravaris, C. L. (1971). Blood monoamine oxidase levels in pregnancy and during the menstrual cycle. *Journal of Psychosomatic Research, 15,* 215–20.

Ginsburg, J., Swinhoe, J., and O'Reilly, B. (1981). Cardiovascular responses during the menopausal hot flush. *British Journal of Obstetrics and Gynecology, 88,* 925–30.

Giugliano, D., Torella, R., Sgambato, S., and D'onofrio, F. (1979). Effects of alpha and beta adrenergic inhibition and somatostatin on plasma glucose, free fatty acids, insulin, glucagon, and growth hormone responses to prostaglandin E_1 in man. *Journal of Clinical Endocrinology and Metabolism, 48,* 302–8.

Goldman, J. A., and Eckerling, B. (1970). Blood glucose levels and glucose tolerance in women with subclinical diabetes receiving oral contraceptives. *American Journal of Obstetrics and Gynecology, 107,* 325–26.

Golub, S. (1976a). The magnitude of premenstrual anxiety and depression. *Psychosomatic Medicine, 38,* 4–12.

——— (1976b). The effect of premenstrual anxiety and depression on cognitive function. *Journal of Personality and Social Psychology, 34,* 99–104.

——— (1981). Sex differences in attitudes and beliefs regarding menstruation. In P. Komnenich, M. McSweeney, J. A. Noack, and N. Elder (Eds.), *The Menstrual Cycle, Volume 2: Research and Implications for Women's Health.* New York: Springer Publishing.

Golub, L. J., Menduke, H., and Conly, S. S. (1965). Weight changes in college women during the menstrual cycle. *American Journal of Obstetrics and Gynecology, 91,* 89–94.

Golub, S., and Narrington, M. (1981). Premenstrual and menstrual mood changes in adolescent women. *Journal of Personality and Social Psychology, 41,* 961–65.

Gough, E. D., and Dyer, D. C. (1971). Responses of isolated human uterine arteries to vasoactive drugs. *American Journal of Obstetrics and Gynecology, 110,* 625–29.

Gough, H. G. (1975). Personality factors related to reported severity of menstrual distress. *Journal of Abnormal Psychology, 84,* 59–64.

Gottschalk, L. A., Kaplan, S. M., Gleser, G. C., and Wingest, C. M. (1962). Variations in magnitude of emotion: A method applied to anxiety and hostility during phases of the menstrual cycle. *Psychosomatic Medicine, 24,* 300–11.

Graham, E. A. (1980). Cognition as related to menstrual cycle phase and estrogen level. In A. J. Dan, E. A. Graham, and C. P. Beecher (Eds.), *The Menstrual Cycle, Volume 1: A Synthesis of Interdisciplinary Research.* New York: Springer Publishing.

Grant, E. C. C., and Mears, E. (1967). Mental effects of oral contraceptive. *Lancet,* October, 945–46.

Grant, E. C. G., and Pryse-Davies, J. (1968). Effect of oral contraceptives on depressive mood changes and on endometrial monoamine oxidase and phosphates. *British Medical Journal, 3,* 777–80.

Gray, L. A., Christopherson, W. M., and Hoover, R. N. (1977). Estrogens and endometrial carcinoma. *Obstetrics and Gynecology, 49,* 385–89.

Gray, M. J., Strausfeld, K. S., Watanabe, M., Sims, E. A. H., and Solomon, S. (1968). Aldosterone secretory rates in the normal menstruating cycle. *Journal of Clinical Endocrinology and Metabolism, 28,* 1269–75.

Green, K., and Hagenfeldt, K. (1975). Prostaglandins in the human endometrium. *American Journal of Obstetrics and Gynecology, 122,* 611–14.

Greene, J. G. (1976). A factor analytic study of climacteric symptoms. *Journal of Psychosomatic Research, 20,* 425–30.

Greene, J. G., and Cooke, D. J. (1980). Life stress and symptoms at the climacterium. *British Journal of Psychiatry, 136,* 486–91.

Greene, R., and Dalton, K. (1953). The premenstrual syndrome. *British Medical Journal,* May, 1007–14.

Greenwald, P., Caputo, T. A., and Wolfgang, P. E. (1977). Endometrial cancer after menopausal use of estrogens. *Obstetrics and Gynecology, 50,* 239–43.

Gregory, B. A. J. C. (1957). The menstrual cycle and its disorders in psychiatric patients: Review of the literature. *Journal of Psychosomatic Research, 2,* 61–79.

Greiss, F. C. (1972). Differential reactivity of the myoendometrial and placental vasculatures: Adrenergic responses. *American Journal of Obstetrics and Gynecology, 112,* 20–30.

Greiss, F. C., and Anderson, S. G. (1970). Effect of ovarian hormones on the uterinevascular bed. *American Journal of Obstetrics and Gynecology, 107,* 829–36.

Grodin, J. M., Siiteri, P. K., and MacDonald, P. C. (1973). Source of estrogen production in postmenopausal women. *Journal of Clinical Endocrinology and Metabolism, 36,* 207–14.

Gruba, G. H., and Rohrbaugh, M. (1975). MMPI correlates of menstrual distress. *Psychosomatic Medicine, 37,* 265–73.

Hackmann, E., Wirz-Justice, W., and Lichtsteiner, M. (1973). The uptake of dopamine and serotonin in rat brain during progesterone decline. *Psychopharmacology, 32,* 183–91.

Hain, J. D., Linton, P. H., Eber, H. W., and Chapman, M. M. (1970). Menstrual irregularity, symptoms and personality. *Journal of Psychosomatic Research, 14,* 81–87.

Halbert, D. R., Demers, L. M., Fontana, J., and Jones, D. E. (1975). Prostaglandin levels inendometrial jet wash specimens in patients with dysmenorrhea before and after indomethacin therapy. *Prostaglandins*, 10, 1047–56.

Halbreich, U., Ben-David, M., Assall, M., and Bornstein. R. (1976). Serum-prolactin in women with premenstrual syndrome. *Lancet*, September, 645–56.

Halbreich, U., and Kas, D. (1977). Variations in the Taylor MAS of women with premenstrual syndrome. *Journal of Psychosomatic Research*, 21, 391–93.

Hall, R., Anderson, J., Smart, G. A., and Besser, M. (1974). *Fundamentals of Clinical Endocrinology* (2nd ed.). London: Pitman Medical.

Hamanaka, Y., Manabe, H., Tanaka, H., Monden, Y., Uozumi, T., and Matsumoto, K. (1970). Effects of surgery on plasma levels of cortisol, corticosterone, and non-protein-bound-cortisol. *Acta Endocrinologica*, 64, 439–51.

Hamburg, D. A. (1966). Effects of progesterone on behavior. In R. Levine (Ed.), *Endocrines and the Central Nervous System*. Baltimore, Md.: Williams and Wilkins.

Hammond, C. B., Jelovsek, F. R., Lee, K. L., Creasman, W. T., and Parker, R. T. (1979). Effects of long-term estrogen replacement therapy. II. Neoplasia. *American Journal of Obstetrics and Gynecology*, 133, 537–47.

Hammond, C. B., and Ory, S. J. (1982). Endocrine problems in the menopause. *Clinical Obstetrics and Gynecology*, 25, 19–38.

Hansen, M. K., and Secher, N. J. (1975). Beta-receptor stimulation in essential dysmenorrhea. *American Journal of Obstetrics and Gynecology*, 121, 566–67.

Hanson, F. W., Izu, A., and Henzl, M. R. (1978). Naproxen sodium in dysmenorrhea: Its influence in allowing continuation of work–school activities. *Obstetrics and Gynecology*, 52, 583–87.

Hanson, J. D., Larson, M. E., and Snowdon, C. T. (1976). The effects of control over high intensity noise on plasma cortisol levels in Rhesus monkeys. *Behavioral Biology*, 16, 333–40.

Hargrove, J. L., Nesbitt, D., Gaspar, M. J., and Ellis, L. C. (1976). Indomethacin induces rat uterine contractions in vitro and alters reactivity to calcium and acetylcholine. *American Journal of Obstetrics and Gynecology, 124,* 25–29.

Hemsell, D. L., Grodin, J. M., Brenner, P. F., Siiteri, P. K., and MacDonald, P. C. (1974). Plasma precursors of estrogen. II. Correlation of extent of conversion of plasma androstenedione to estrone with age. *Journal of Clinical Endocrinology and Metabolism, 38,* 476–79.

Heneson, N. (1984). The selling of PMS. *Science 84,* May, 66–71.

Hendricks, C. H. (1966). Characteristics of the nonpregnant human uterus. *American Journal of Obstetrics and Gynecology, 96,* 824–43.

Henrik, E. (1982). Neuroendocrine mechanisms of reproductive aging in women and female rats. In A. M. Voda, M. Dinnerstein, and S. R. O'Connell (Eds.), *Changing Perspectives on Menopause.* Austin: University of Texas Press.

Henzl, M. R., Buttram, V., Segre, E. J., and Bessler, S. (1977). The treatment of dysmenorrhea with naproxen sodium: A report on two independent double-blind trials. *American Journal of Obstetrics and Gynecology, 127,* 818–23.

Henzl, M. R., Moyer, D. L., Townsend, D., Valand, R. S., and Segre, E. J. (1973). Quantitation of the estrogenic effects of mestranol on human endometrium and vaginal mucosa. *American Journal of Obstetrics and Gynecology, 115,* 401–6.

Henzl, M. R., Ortega-Herrera, E., Rodriquez, C., and Izu, A. (1979). Anaprox in dysmenorrhea: Reduction of pain and intrauterine pressure. *American Journal of Obstetrics and Gynecology, 135,* 455–60.

Herzberg, B. (1971). Body composition and premenstrual tension. *Journal of Psychosomatic Research, 15,* 251–57.

Hillier, K., Dutton, A., Corker, C. S., Singer, A., and Embrey, M. P. (1972). Plasma steroid and lutenizing hormone levels during prostaglandin F_{2a} administration in the luteal phase of menstrual cycle. *British Medical Journal, 4,* 333–36.

Hirt, M., Kurtz, R., and Ross, W. D. (1967). The relationship between dysmenorrhea and selected personality variables. *Psychosomatics, 8,* 350–53.

Hoff, J. D., Lasley, B. L., and Yen, S. S. C. (1979). The functional relationship between priming and releasing actions of lutenizing hormone-releasing hormone. *Journal of Clinical Endocrinology and Metabolism, 49,* 8–11.

Hoff, J. D., Quigley, M. E., and Yen, S. S. C. (1983). Hormonal dynamics at midcycle: A reevaluation. *Journal of Clinical Endrocrinology and Metabolism, 57,* 792–96.

Hofmann, C. E., Rao, C. V., Barrows, G. H., and Sanfilippo, J. S. (1983). Topography of human uterine prostaglandin E and F_{2a} receptors and their profiles during pathological state. *Journal of Clinical Endocrinology and Metabolism, 4,* 302–12.

Holding, T. A., and Minkoff, K. (1973). Parasuicide and the menstrual cycle. *Journal of Psychosomatic Research, 17,* 365–68.

Hoover, R., Gray, L. A., Cole, P., MacMahan, B. (1976). Menopausal estrogens and breast cancer. *New England Journal of Medicine, 295,* 401–5.

Hopson, J., and Rosenfeld, A. (1984). PMS: Puzzling monthly symptoms. *Psychology Today,* August, 30–35.

Hossain, M., Smith, D. A., and Nordin, B. E. C. (1970). Parathyroid activity and postmenopausal osteoporosis. *Lancet,* April, 809–11.

Hulka, B. S., Chambless, L. E., Deubner, D. C., and Wilkinson, W. E. (1982). Breast cancer and estrogen replacement therapy. *American Journal of Obstetrics and Gynecology, 143,* 638–44.

Hunter, D. J. S. (1976). Oophorectomy and the surgical menopause. In R. J. Beard (Ed.), *The Menopause: A Guide to Current Research & Practice.* Baltimore, Md.: University Park Press.

Hunter, D. J. S., Anderson, A. B. M., and Haddon, M. (1979). Changes in coagulation factors in postmenopausal women on ethinyl oestradiol. *British Journal of Obstetrics and Gynecology, 86,* 488–90.

Hunter, D. J. S., Julier, D., Franklin, M., and Green, E. (1977). Plasma levels of estrogen, lutenizing hormone, and follicle stimulating hormone following castration and estradiol implant. *Obstetrics and Gynecology, 49,* 180–85.

Huseman, C. A., Kugler, J. A., and Schneider, I. G. (1980). Mechanism of dopaminergic suppression of gonadotropin secretion in men. *Journal of Clinical Endocrinology and Metabolism, 51,* 209–14.

Hutt, Mychalkiw, F. W., and Hughes, M. (1980). Perceptual-motor performance during the menstrual cycle. *Hormones and Behavior, 14*, 116–25.

Hutton, J. D., Jacobs, H. S., Murray, M. A. F., and James, V. H. T. (1978). Relation between plasma oestrone and oestradiol and climacteric symptoms. *Lancet*, April, 678–81.

Israel, S. (1953). The clinical pattern and etiology of premenstrual tension. *International Record of Medicine, 166*, 469–74.

—— (1967). *Diagnosis and Treatment of Menstrual Disorders and Sterility.* New York: Harper & Row.

Ivey, M. E., and Bardwick, M. J. (1968). Patterns of affective fluctuation in the menstrual cycle. *Psychosomatic Medicine, 30*, 336–45.

Jacobs, B. R., Suchocki, S., and Smith, R. G. (1980). Evidence for a human ovarian progesterone receptor. *American Journal of Obstetrics and Gynecology, 138*, 332–36.

Janowsky, D. S., Berens, S. C., and Davis, J. M. (1973). Correlations between mood, weight, and electrolytes during the menstrual cycle: A renin–angiotensin–aldosterone hypothesis of premenstrual tension. *Psychosomatic Medicine, 35*, 143–154.

Janowsky, D. S., and Davis, J. M. (1970). Progesterone–estrogen effects on uptake and release of norepinephrine by synaptosomes. *Life Sciences, 9*, 525–31.

Jeffcoate, T. N. A. (1960). Drugs for menopausal symptoms. *British Medical Journal*, January, 340–42.

Jensen, G. F., Christiansen, C., and Transbol, I. B. (1982). Fracture frequency and bone preservation in postmenopausal women treated with estrogen. *Obstetrics and Gynecology, 60*, 493–96.

Jern, H. Z. (1973). *Hormone therapy of the menopause and aging.* Springfield, Ill.: Charles C Thomas.

Jewelewicz, R., Cantor, B., Dyrenfurth, I., Warren, M. P., and Vande Wiele, R. L. (1972). Intravenous infusion of prostaglandin F_{2a} in the mid-luteal phase of the normal menstrual cycle. *Prostaglandins, 7*, 2387–88.

Jordan, V. C., and Pokoly, T. B. (1977). Steroid and prostaglandin relations during the menstrual cycle. *Obstetrics and Gynecology, 49*, 449–53.

Judd, H. L., Davidson, B. J., Frumar, A. M., Shamonki, I. M., and Logasse, L. D. (1982). Origin of serum estradiol in postmenopausal women. *Obstetrics and Gynecology, 59,* 680–86.

Judd, H. L., Davidson, B. J., Frumar, A. M., Shamonki, I. M., Logasse, L. D., and Ballon, S. C. (1980). Serum androgens and estrogens in postmenopausal women with and without endometrial cancer. *American Journal of Obstetrics and Gynecology, 136,* 859–66.

Judd, H. L., Judd, G. E., Lucas, W. E., and Yen, S. S. C. (1974). Endocrine function of the postmenopausal ovary: Concentration of androgens and estrogens in ovarian and peripheral vein blood. *Journal of Clinical Endocrinology and Metabolism, 39,* 1020–24.

Judd, H. L., Lucas, W. E., and Yen, S. S. C. (1976). Serum 17B-estradiol and estrone levels in postmenopausal women with and without endometrial cancer. *Journal of Clinical Endocrinology and Metabolism, 43,* 272–78.

Judd, S. J., Rakoff, J. S., and Yen, S. S. C. (1978). Inhibition of gonadotropin and prolactin release by dopamine: Effect of endogenous estradiol levels. *Journal of Clinical Endocrinology and Metabolism, 47,* 494–98.

Judd, S. J., Rigg, L. A., and Yen, S. S. C. (1979). The effects of ovariectomy and estrogen treatment on the dopamine inhibition of gonadotropin and prolactin release. *Journal of Clinical Endocrinology and Metabolism, 49,* 182–84.

Kapan, S. J., Vagenakis, A., and Braverman, L. (1980). Failure of a serotonergic receptor-blocking drug to change the twenty-four-hour luteinizing hormone secretory pattern in women. *Journal of Clinical Endocrinology and Metabolism, 51,* 302–6.

Kaplan, A. (1964). *The Conduct of Inquiry.* San Francisco: Chandler.

Karim, S. M., and Hillier, K. (1973). The role of prostaglandins in myometrial contraction. In J. B. Josimovich (Ed.), *Uterine Contraction—Side Effects of Steroidal Contraceptives.* New York: Wiley.

Kashiwagi, T., McClure, J. N., and Wetzel, R. D. (1976). Premenstrual affective syndrome and psychiatric disorder. *Diseases of the Nervous System, 37,* 116–19.

Katra, S. P., and McCann, S. M. (1974). Effects of drugs modifying catecholamine synthesis on plasma LH and ovulation in the rat. *Neuroendocrinology, 15,* 79–91.

Katz, F. H., and Romfh, P. (1972). Plasma aldosterone and renin activity during the menstrual cycle. *Journal of Clinical Endocrinology and Metabolism, 34,* 819–21.

Kaufman, S. A. (1967). Limited relationship of maturation index to estrogen therapy for menopausal symptoms. *Obstetrics and Gynecology, 54,* 399–407.

Kerin, J. F., Edmonds, D. K., Warnes, G. M., Cox, L. W., Seamark, F. F., Mathews, C. D., Young, G. B., and Baird, D. T. (1981). Morphological and functional relations of graafian follicle growth to ovulation in women using ultrasonic laparoscopic and biochemical measurements. *British Journal of Obstetrics and Gynecology, 88,* 81–90.

King, R. J. B., Whitehead, M. I., Campbell, S., and Minardi, J. (1978). Effects of estrogens and progestogens on the biochemistry of the postmenopausal endometrium. In I. D. Cooke (Ed.), *The Menopause: A Guide to Current Research and Practice.* Baltimore, Md.: University Park Press.

Kirton, K. T. (1973). Biochemical effects of prostaglandins as they might relate to uterine contraction. In J. B. Josimovich (Ed.), *Uterine Contraction—Side Effects of Steroidal Contraceptives.* New York: Wiley.

Kistner, R. W. (1976). Estrogens and endometrial cancer: An editorial. *Obstetrics and Gynecology, 48,* 479–82.

Klaiber, E. L., Broverman, D. M., Vogel, W., Kobayashi, Y., and Moriarity, D. (1972). Effects of estrogen therapy on plasma MAO activity and EEG driving response of depressed women. *American Journal of Psychiatry, 128,* 1492–98.

Klaiber, E. L., Kobayashi, Y., Broverman, D. M., and Hall, F. (1971). Plasma monoamine oxidase activity in regularly menstruating women and in amenorrheic women receiving cyclic treatment with estrogens and a progestin. *Journal of Clinical Endocrinology and Metabolism, 33,* 630–38.

Koeske, R. K. (1980). Theoretical perspectives on menstrual cycle research: The relevance of attributional approaches for the perception and explanation of premenstrual emotionality. In A. J. Dan, E. A. Graham, and C. P. Beecher (Eds.), *The Menstrual Cycle, Volume 1: A Synthesis of Interdisciplinary Research.* New York: Springer Publishing.

—— (1982). Toward a biosocial paradigm for menopausal research: Lessons and contributions from behavioral sciences. In A. Voda, M. Dinnerstein, and S. R. O'Connell (Eds.), *Changing Perspectives on Menopause.* Austin: University of Texas Press.

Koeske, R. D., and Koeske, G. F. (1975). An attributional approach to moods and the menstrual cycle. *Journal of Personality and Social Psychology, 31,* 473–78.

Kopell, B. S., Lunde, D. T., Clayton, R. B., and Moos, R. H. (1969). Variations in some measures of arousal during the menstrual cycle. *Journal of Nervous and Mental Disorders, 148,* 180–87.

Krieger, D. T. (1980). The hypothalamus and neuroendocrinology. In D. T. Krieger and J. C. Hughes (Eds.), *Neuroendocrinology.* Sunderland, Mass.: Sinauer Associates, Inc.

Kroger, W. S., and Freed, S. C. (1943). The psychosomatic treatment of functional dysmenorrhea by hypnosis. *American Journal of Obstetrics and Gynecology, 46,* 817–22.

Kudrow, L. (1978). Current aspects of migraine headache. *Psychosomatics,* 48–57.

Kupperman, H. S., Blatt, M. H. G., Wiesbader, H., and Filler, W. (1953). Comparative clinical evaluation of estrogenic preparations by the menopausal and amenorrheal indices. *Journal of Clinical Endocrinology and Metabolism, 13,* 688–701.

Kitner, S. J., and Brown, W. L. (1972). Types of oral contraceptives, depression, and premenstrual symptoms. *Journal of Nervous and Mental Disorders, 155,* 153–62.

Lachelin, G. C. L., Leblanc, H., and Yen, S. S. C. (1977). The inhibitory effect of dopamine agonists on LH release in women. *Journal of Clinical Endocrinology and Metabolism, 44,* 728–32.

Lahmeyer, H. W., Miller, M., and DeLeon-Jones, F. (1982). Anxiety and mood fluctuation during the normal menstrual cycle. *Psychosomatic Medicine, 44,* 183–94.

Laidlow, J. C., Ruse, J. L., and Gornall, A. G. (1962). The influence of estrogen and progesterone on aldosterone excretion. *Journal of Clinical Endocrinology and Metabolism, 22,* 161–71.

Landau, R. L., and Lugibihl, K. (1958). Inhibition of the sodium-retaining influence of aldosterone by progesterone. *Journal of Clinical Endocrinology and Metabolism, 18,* 1236–45.

Langer, G. H., and Sachar, E. J. (1977). Dopaminergic factors in human prolactin regulation: Effects of neuroleptics and dopamine. *Psychoneuroendocrinology*, 2, 373–78.

Langer, G., Sachar, E. J., Gruen, P. H., and Halpern, F. S. (1977a). Human prolactin responses to neuroleptic drugs correlate with antischizophrenic potency. *Nature*, 266, 639–40.

Langer, G., Sachar, E. J., Halpern, F. S., Gruen, P. H., and Solomon, M. (1977b). The prolactin response to neuroleptic drugs. A test of dopaminergic blockage: Neuronendocrine studies in normal men. *Journal of Clinical Endocrinology and Metabolism*, 45, 996–1002.

Laragh, J. H. (1976). Oral contraceptive-induced hypertension—Nine years later. *American Journal of Obstetrics and Gynecology*, 126, 141–47.

Larkin, R. M., VanOrder, D. E., Poulson, A. M., and Scott, J. R. (1979). Dysmenorrhea: Treatment with an antiprostaglandin. *Obstetrics and Gynecology*, 54, 456–60.

Larsson-Cohn, U. (1975). Oral contraceptives and vitamins: A review. *American Journal of Obstetrics and Gynecology*, 121, 84–90.

Larsson-Cohn, U., Johansson, E. D. B., Kagedal, B., and Wallentin, L. (1978). Serum FSH, LH, and oestrone levels in postmenopausal patients on eostrogen therapy. *British Journal of Obstetrics and Gynecology*, 85, 367–72.

LaTorre, R. A. (1974). Estradiol inhibition of catecholaminergic eating in the castrated female rat. *Biological Psychiatry*, 8, 337–41.

Laufer, L. R., Erlik, Y., Meldrum, D. R., and Judd, H. L. (1982). Effect of clonidine on hot flashes in postmenopausal women. *Obstetrics and Gynecology*, 60, 583–86.

Lawoyin, S., Zerwekh, J. E., Glass, K., and Pak, C. Y. C. (1980). Ability of 25-hydroxyvitamin D therapy to augment serum 1,25- and 24,25-dyhydroxy-vitamin D in postmenopausal osteoporosis. *Journal of Clinical Endocrinology and Metabolism*, 50, 593–96.

Leblanc, H., Lachelin, G. C. L., Abu-fadil, S., and Yen, S. S. C. (1976). Effects of dopamine infusion on pituitary hormone secretion in humans. *Journal of Clinical Endocrinology and Metabolism*, 43, 668–74.

Leblanc, H., and Yen, S. S. C. (1976). The effect of L-dopa and chlorpromazine on prolactin and growth hormone secretion in normal women. *American Journal of Obstetrics and Gynecology*, 126, 162–64.

Leebaw, W. F., Lee, L. A., and Woolf, P. D. (1978). Dopamine affects basal and augmented pituitary hormone secretion. *Journal of Clinical Endocrinology and Metabolism, 47*, 480–87.

Lehrer, D. N. (1965). Effect of some spasmolytic drugs on the isolated human myometrium. *Journal of Pharmacology, 17*, 584–88.

Lennane, K. J., and Lennane, R. J. (1973). Alleged psychogenic disorders in women: A possible manifestation of sexual prejudice. *New England Journal of Medicine, ii*, 288–92.

Levitt, E. E., and Lubin, B. (1967). Some personality factors associated with menstrual attitudes. *Journal of Psychosomatic Research, 11*, 267–70.

Levy, C., Robel, P., Gautray, J. P., DeBrux, J., Verma, U., Descomps, B., Baulieru, E. E., and Eychenne, B. (1980). Estradiol and progesterone receptors in human endometrium: Normal and abnormal menstrual cycles and early pregnancy. *American Journal of Obstetrics and Gynecology, 136*, 646–51.

Lightman, S. L., Jacobs, H. S., and Maguire, A. K. (1982), Down-regulation of gonadotropin secretion in postmenopausal women by a superactive LHRH analogue: Lack of effect of menopausal flushing. *British Journal of Obstetrics and Gynecology, 89*, 977–80.

Lightman, S. L., Jacobs, H. S., Maguire, A. K., McGarrick, G., and Jeffcoate, S. L. (1981). Climacteric flushing: Clinical and endocrine response to infusion of naloxone. *British Journal of Obstetrics and Gynecology, 88*, 919–24.

Lin, T., SoBosita, J. L., Brar, H. K., and Roblete, B. V. (1973). Clinical and cytologic responses of postmenopausal women to estrogen. *Obstetrics and Gynecology, 41*, 97–107.

Lind, T. (1978). A prospective controlled trial of six forms of hormone replacement therapy after the menopause. In I. D. Cooke (Ed.), *The Role of Estrogen/Progesterone in the Management of Menopause.* Baltimore, Md.: University Park Press.

Lind, T., Cameron, E. C., Hunter, W. M., Leon, C., Moran, P. F., Oxley, A., Gerrard, J., and Lind, U. C. G. (1979). A prospective, controlled trial of six forms of hormone replacement therapy given to postmenopausal women. *British Journal of Obstetrics and Gynecology, 86*, Supplement 3, 1–29.

Lindsay, R., Hart, D. M., Maclean, H. A., Garwood, J., Aitken, J. M., Clark, A. C., and Coutts, J. R. T. (1978). In I. D. Cooke (Ed.), *The Role of*

Estrogen/Progesterone in the Management of Menopause. Baltimore, Md.: University Park Press.

Little, B. C., and Zahn, T. P. (1974). Changes in mood and autonomic functioning during the menstrual cycle. Psychophysiology, 11, 579–90.

Lobo, R. A., Goebelsmann, U., Brenner, P. F., and Mishell, D. R. (1982). The effects of estrogen on adrenal androgens in oophorectomized women. American Journal of Obstetrics and Gynecology, 142, 471–78.

Longcope, C., Hunter, R., and Franz, C. (1980). Steroid secretion by the postmenopausal ovary. American Journal of Obstetrics and Gynecology, 138, 564–68.

Lucas, W. E., and Yen, S. S. C. (1979). A study of endocrine and metabolic variables in postmenopausal women with endometrial carcinoma. American Journal of Obstetrics and Gynecology, 134, 180–86.

Lundstrom, V., and Green, K. (1978). Endogenous levels of prostaglandin F_{2a} and its main metabolites in plasma and endometrium of normal and dysmenorrheic women. American Journal of Obstetrics and Gynecology, 30, 640–46.

Lundstrom, V., Green, K., and Wiquist, N. (1976). Prostaglandins, indomethacin and dysmenorrhea. Prostaglandins, 11, 893–904.

Lyrenas, S., Karlstrom, K., Backstrom, T., and von Schoultz, B. (1981). A comparison of serum oestrogen levels after percutaneous and oral administration of oestradiol-17B. British Journal of Obstetrics and Gynecology, 88, 181–87.

Maathius, J. B. (1978). Cyclic changes in the concentration of prostaglandin F_{2a} in human uterine flushings. British Journal of Obstetrics and Gynecology, 85, 207–10.

MacKinnon, I. L., MacKinnon, P. C. D., and Thomson, A. D. (1959). Lethal hazards of the luteal phase of the menstrual cycle. British Medical Journal, April, 1015–17.

Maddock, J. (1978). Gonadal and pituitary hormone profiles in perimenopausal patients. In I. D. Cooke (Ed.), The Role of Estrogen/Progesterone in the Management of the Menopause. Baltimore, Md.: University Park Press.

Mahajan, D. K., Billiar, R. B., Jassani, M., and Little, A. B. (1978). Ethinyl estradiol administration and plasma steroid concentration in ovariectomized women. *American Journal of Obstetrics and Gynecology*, *130*, 398–402.

Maier, S. F., Sherman, F. E., Lewis, J. W., Terman, G. W., and Liebeskind, J. C. (1983). The opioid/nonopioid nature of stress-induced analgesia and learned helplessness. *Journal of Experimental Psychology: Animal Behavior Processes*, *9*, 80–90.

Mandel, F. P., Geola, F. L., Lu, J. K., Eggena, P., Sambhi, M. P., Hershman, J. M., and Judd, H. L. (1982). Biologic effects of various doses of ethinyl estradiol in postmenopausal women. *Obstetrics and Gynecology*, *59*, 673–79.

Mandel. F. P., Geola, F. L., Meldrum, D. R., Lu, J. H. K., Eggena, P., Sambhi, M. P., Hershman, J. M., and Judd, H. L. (1983). Biological effects of various doses of vaginally administered conjugated equine estrogens in postmenopausal women. *Journal of Clinical Endocrinology and Metabolism*, *57*, 133–39.

Mandell, A. J., and Mandell, M. P. (1967). Suicide and the menstrual cycle. *American Medical Association Journal*, *200*, 792–93.

Maoz, B., Dowty, N., Antonovsky, A., and Wijsenbeek, H. (1970). Female attitudes to menopause. *Social Psychiatry*, *5*, 35–40.

March, C. M., Goebelsmann, U., Nakamura, R. M., and Mishell, D. R. (1979). Roles of estradiol and progesterone in eliciting the midcycle luteinizing hormone and follicle-stimulating hormone surges. *Journal of Clinical Endocrinology and Metabolism*, *49*, 507–13.

Marinari, K., Leshner, A. I., and Doyle, M. P. (1976). Menstrual cycle status and adrenocortical reactivity to psychological stress. *Psychoneuroendocrinology*, *1*, 213–18.

Markum, R. A. (1976). Assessment of reliability of and the effect of neutral instructions on the symptom ratings on the Moos Menstrual Distress Questionnaire. *Psychosomatic Medicine*, *38*, 163–72.

Maroulis, G. B., and Abraham, G. E. (1976). Ovarian and adrenal contributions to peripheral steroid levels in postmenopausal women. *Obstetrics and Gynecology*, *48*, 150–54.

Marshall, J. (1963). Thermal changes in the normal menstrual cycle. *British Medical Journal*, January, 102–4.

Martin, P. L., Burnier, A. M., and Greaney, M. O. (1972). Oral menopausal therapy using 17-B micronized estradiol. *Obstetrics and Gynecology*, *39*, 771–74.

Martin, P. L., Burnier, A. M., Segre, E. J., and Huix, F. J. (1971). Graded sequential therapy in the menopause: A double-blind study. American Journal of Obstetrics and Gynecology, 111, 178–86.

Maslar, I. A., and Riddick, D. H. (1979). Prolactin production by human endometrium during the normal menstrual cycle. American Journal of Obstetrics and Gynecology, 135, 751–54.

Mason, J. W. (1975). Psychologic stress and endocrine function. In E. J. Sachar (Ed.), Topics in Psychoendocrinology. New York: Grune and Stratton.

Mason, J. W., Hartley, H., Kotchen, T. A., Mougey, E. H., Ricketts, P. T., and Jones, L. G. (1973). Plasma cortisol and norepinephrine responses in anticipation of muscular exercise. Psychosomatic Medicine, 35, 406–14.

Mason, J. W., Maher, J. T., Hartley, L. H., Maugey, E. H., Perlow, M. J., and Jones, L. G. (1976). Selectivity of corticosteroid and catecholamine responses to various natural stimuli, In G. Serban (Ed.), Psychopathology of Human Adaptation. New York: Plenum.

Matthews, K. A., and Carra, J. (1982). Suppression of menstrual distress symptoms: A study of Type A behavior. Personality and Social Psychological Bulletin, 8, 146–51.

Mattingly, R. F., and Huang, W. Y. (1969). Steroidogenesis of the menopausal and postmenopausal ovary. American Journal of Obstetrics and Gynecology, 103, 679–90.

Mattsson, B., and Schoultz, B. (1974). A comparison between lithium, placebo, and a diuretic in premenstrual tension. Acta Psychiatrica Scandinavia, Supplement 255, 75–84.

May, R. R. (1976). Mood shifts and the menstrual cycle. Journal of Psychosomatic Research, 20, 125–30.

McClintock, M. K. (1981). Major gaps in menstrual cycle research: Behavioral and psychological controls in a biological context. In P. Komnenich, M. McSweeney, J. A. Noack, and N. Elder, The Menstrual Cycle, Volume 2: Research and Implications for Women's Health. New York: Springer Publishing.

McKinlay, S. M., and Jeffreys, M. (1974). The menopausal syndrome. British Journal of Preventative and Social Medicine, 28, 108–15.

McLaughlin, M. K., Brennan, S. C., and Chez, R. A. (1978). Effects of indomethacin on sheep uteroplacental circulations and sensitivity to angiotensin II. *American Journal of Obstetrics and Gynecology, 132,* 430–35.

Meldrum, D. R., Davidson, B. J., Tataryn, I. V., and Judd, H. L. (1981a). Changes in circulating steroids with aging in postmenopausal women. *Obstetrics and Gynecology, 57,* 624–28.

Meldrum, D. R., Erlik, Y., Lu, J. K. H., and Judd, H. L. (1981b). Objectively recorded hot flashes in patients with pituitary insufficiency. *Journal of Clinical Endocrinology and Metabolism, 52,* 684–87.

Meldrum, D. R., Shamonki, I. M., Frumar, A. M., Tataryn, I. V., Chang, R. J., and Judd, H. L. (1979). Elevations in skin temperature of the finger as an objective index of postmenopausal hot flashes: Standardization of the technique. *American Journal of Obstetrics and Gynecology, 135,* 713–17.

Meldrum, D. R., Tataryn, I. V., Frumar, A. M., Erlik, Y., Lu, K. H., and Judd, H. L. (1980). Gonadotropins, estrogens and adrenal steroids during the menopausal hot flash. *Journal of Clinical Endocrinology and Metabolism, 50,* 685–89.

Michelakis, A. M., Stant, E. G., and Brill, A. B. (1971). Sodium space and electrolyte excretion during the menstrual cycle. *American Journal of Obstetrics and Gynecology, 109,* 150–54.

Michelakis, A. M., Yoshida, H., and Dormois, J. C. (1975). Plasma renin activity and plasma aldosterone during the normal menstrual cycle. *American Journal of Obstetrics and Gynecology, 123,* 724–26.

Miller, N. E., and Weiss, J. M. (1969). Effects of somatic or visceral responses to punishment. In B. A. Campbell and R. M. Church (Eds.), *Punishment and Aversive Behavior.* New York: Appleton-Century-Crofts.

Miyabo, S., Asato, T., and Mizushima, N. (1977). Prolactin and growth hormone responses to psychological stress in normal and neurotic subjects. *Journal of Clinical Endocrinology and Metabolism, 44,* 947–51.

Moawad, A. H. (1973). The sympathetic nervous system and the uterus. In J. B. Josimovich (Ed.), *Uterine Contraction—Side Effects of Steroidal Contraceptives.* New York: Wiley.

240 / References

Moghissi, K. S., Syner, F. N., and Evans, T. N. (1972). A composite picture of the menstrual cycle. *American Journal of Obstetrics and Gynecology, 114,* 405–16.

Molitch, M. E., Oill, P., and Odell, W. D. (1974). Massive hyperlipemia during estrogen therapy. *Journal of the American Medical Association, 227,* 522–25.

Molnar, G. W. (1981). Menopausal hot flashes: Their cycles and relation to air temperature. *Obstetrics and Gynecology, 57,* 52–55.

Monroe, S. E., Jaffe, R. B., and Midgley, A. T. (1972). Regulation of human gonadotropins. XII. Increase in serum gonadotropins in response to estradiol. *Journal of Clinical Endocrinology and Metabolism, 34,* 342–47.

Moon, Y. S., Leung, P. C. S., Yuen, B. H., and Gomel, V. (1981). Prostaglandin F in human endometriosic tissue. *American Journal of Obstetrics and Gynecology, 141,* 344–45.

Moore, B., Paterson, M. E. L., Sturdee, D. W., and Whitehead, T. P. (1981). The effect of menopausal status and sequential mestranol and norethisterone on serum biochemical profiles. *British Journal of Obstetrics and Gynecology, 88,* 853–58.

Moos, R. H. (1968). The development of a Menstrual Distress Questionnaire. *Psychosomatic Medicine, 30,* 853.

—— (1969). Typology of menstrual cycle symptoms. *American Journal of Obstetrics and Gynecology, 103,* 390–402.

—— (1977). *Menstrual Distress Questionnaire Manual.* Palo Alto, Calif.: Social Ecology Laboratory.

Moos, R. H., Kopell, B. S., Melges, F. T., Yalom, I. D., Lunde, D. T., Clayton, R. B., and Hamburg, D. A. (1969). Fluctuations in symptoms and moods during the menstrual cycle. *Journal of Psychosomatic Research, 13,* 37–44.

Morris, N. M., and Udry, J. R. (1970). Variations in pedometer activity during the menstrual cycle. *Obstetrics and Gynecology, 35,* 199–201.

Morrison, J. C., Martin, D. C., Blair, R. A., Anderson, G. D., Kincheloe, B. W., Bates, G. W., Hendrix, J. W., Rivlin, M. E., Forman, E. K., Propst, M. G., and Needham, R. (1980). The use of medroxyprogesterone acetate for relief of climacteric symptoms. *American Journal of Obstetrics and Gynecology, 138,* 99–104.

Morse, A. R., Hutton, J. D., Murray, M. A. F., and James, V. H. T. (1979). Relation between the karyophyknotic index and plasma oestrogen concentrations after the menopause. *British Journal of Obstetrics and Gynecology*, 86, 981–83.

Morton, J. H. (1950). Premenstrual tension. *American Journal of Obstetrics and Gynecology*, 60, 343–52.

Morton, J. H., Additon, H., Addison, R. G., Hunt, L., and Sullivan, J. J. (1965). A clinical study of premenstrual tension. *American Journal of Obstetrics and Gynecology*, 65, 1182–91.

Mullen, F. G. (1968). The treatment of a case of dysmenorrhea by behavior therapy techniques. *Journal of Nervous and Mental Disease*, 147, 371–76.

Muller, H. (1969). Sex, age, and hyperparathyroidism. *Lancet*, March, 449–50.

Mulley, G., Mitchell, J. R. A., and Tattersall, R. B. (1977). Hot flushes after hypophysectomy. *British Medical Journal*, October, 1062.

Murakami, T., Yamaji, T., and Ohsawa, K. (1976). The effect of ACTH administration on serum estrogens, LH and FSH in the aged. *Journal of Clinical Endocrinology and Metabolism*, 42, 88–90.

Nachtigall, L. E., Nachtigall, R. H., Nachtigall, R. D., and Beckman, E. M. (1979a). Estrogen replacement therapy: A 10-year prospective study in the relationship to osteoporosis. *Obstetrics and Gynecology*, 53, 277–81.

—— (1979b). Estrogen replacement therapy II: A prospective study in the relationship to carcinoma and cardiovascular and metabolic problems. *Obstetrics and Gynecology*, 54, 74–79.

National Dairy Council (1982). Diet and bone health. *Dairy Council Digest*, 53, 25–30.

Natrajan, P. K., Muldoon, T. G., Greenblatt, R. B., and Mahesh, V. B. (1981). Estradiol and progesterone receptors in estrogen-primed endometrium. *American Journal of Obstetrics and Gynecology*, 140, 387–92.

Navratil, J. (1975). The pathogenesis of premenstrual tension. *Activitas Nervosa Superior*, 17, 304–5.

Nesheim, B. I., and Walloe, L. (1976). The use of isoxsuprine in essential dysmenorrhea. *Acta Obstetrica Gynecologia Scandinavia*, 55, 315–16.

Newman, W. P., and Brodows, R. G. (1982). Metabolic effects of prostaglandin E_2 infusion in man: Possible adrenergic mediation. *Journal of Clinical Endocrinology and Metabolism, 55*, 496–501.

Nillius, S. J., and Wise, L. (1970). Effects of oestrogen on serum levels of LH and FSH. *Acta Endocrinologica, 65*, 583–94.

Nisker, J. A., Hammond, G. L., Davidson, B. J., Frumar, A. M., Takaki, N. K., Judd, H. L., and Siiteri, P. K. (1980). Serum sex-hormone-binding-globulin capacity and the percentage of free estradiol in postmenopausal women with and without endometrial carcinoma. *American Journal of Obstetrics and Gynecology, 138*, 637–42.

Noel, G. L., Suh, H. K., Stone, J. G., and Frantz, A. G. (1972). Human prolactin and growth hormone release during surgery and other conditions of stress. *Journal of Clinical Endocrinology and Metabolism, 35*, 840–57.

Nordin, B. E. C. (1971). Clinical significance and pathogenesis of osteoporosis. *British Medical Journal, i*, 571–76.

Notelovitz, M., Kitchens, C. J., Coone, L., McKenzie, L., and Carter, R. (1981). Low-dose oral contraceptive usage and coagulation. *American Journal of Obstetrics and Gynecology, 141*, 71–75.

Notelovitz, M., Kitchens, C. S., Rappaport, V., Coone, L., and Dougherty, M. (1981). Menopausal status associated with increased inhibition of blood coagulation. *American Journal of Obstetrics and Gynecology, 141*, 149–52.

Notelovitz, M., Kitchens, C., Ware, M., Hirschberg, K., and Coone, L. (1983). Combination estrogen and progestogen replacement therapy does not adversely affect coagulation. *Obstetrics and Gynecology, 62*, 596.

Nowaczynski, W., Murakami, T., Richardson, K., and Genest, J. (1978). Increased aldosterone plasma protein binding in women on combined oral contraceptives throughout the menstrual cycle. *Journal of Clinical Endocrinology and Metabolism, 47*, 193–99.

O'Brien, P. M. S., Craven, D., Selby, C., and Symonds, E. M. (1979). Treatment of premenstrual syndrome by spironolactone. *British Journal of Obstetrics and Gynecology, 86*, 142–47.

O'Brien, P. M. S., and Symonds, E. M. (1982). Prolactin levels in the premenstrual syndrome. *British Journal of Obstetrics and Gynecology, 89*, 306–8.

Okamura, H., Okazaki, T., and Nakajima, A. (1974). Effects of neurotransmitters and prostaglandins on human ovarian contractility. *Obstetrics and Gynecology, 44*, 720–26.

Osofsky, J. J., and Seidenberg, R. (1970). Is female menopausal depression inevitable? *Obstetrics and Gynecology, 36*, 611–15.

Ostergard, D. R., Parlow, A. F., and Townsend, D. E. (1970). Acute effect of castration on serum FSH and LH in the adult woman. *Journal of Clinical Endocrinology and Metabolism, 31*, 43–47.

Paige, K. E. (1971). Effects of oral contraceptives on affective fluctuations associated with the menstrual cycle. *Psychosomatic Medicine, 33*, 515–37.

___ (1973). Women learn to sing the menstrual blues. *Psychology Today*, September, 41–46.

Palmblad, J., Blomback, M., Egberg, N., Froberg, J., Karlsson, C. G., and Levi, L. (1977). Experimentally induced stress in man: Effects on blood coagulation and fibrinolysis. *Journal of Psychosomatic Research, 21*, 87–92.

Parker, C. R., Winkel, C. A., Rush, J., Porter, J. C., and MacDonald, P. C. (1981). Plasma concentrations of 11-deoxycorticosterone in women during the menstrual cycle. *Obstetrics and Gynecology, 58*, 26–30.

Parlee, M. B. (1973). The premenstrual syndrome. *Psychological Bulletin, 80*, 454–65.

___ (1974). Stereotypic beliefs about menstruation: A methodological note on the Moos Menstrual Distress Questionnaire and some new data. *Psychosomatic Medicine, 36*, 229–40.

___ (1980). Positive changes in moods and activation levels during the menstrual cycle in experimentally naive subjects. In A. J. Dan, E. A. Graham, and C. P. Beecher (Eds.), *The Menstrual Cycle, Volume 1: A Synthesis of Interdisciplinary Research*. New York: Springer Publishing.

Paterson, M. E. L. (1982). A randomized double-blind cross-over trial into the effect of norethisterone on climacteric symptoms and biochemical profiles. *British Journal of Obstetrics and Gynecology, 89*, 464–72.

Paterson, M. E. L., Sturdee, D. W., Moore, B., and Whitehead, T. P. (1979). The effect of menopausal status and sequential mestranol and norethisterone on serum cholesterol, triglyceride, and electrophoretic lipoprotein patterns. *British Journal of Obstetrics and Gynecology, 86,* 810–15.

——— (1980). The effect of various regimens of hormone therapy on serum cholesterol and triglyceride concentrations in postmenopausal women. *British Journal of Obstetrics and Gynecology, 87,* 552–60.

Patkai, P., Johannson, G., and Post, B. (1974). Mood alertness and sympathetic-adrenal medullary activity during the menstrual cycle. *Psychosomatic Medicine, 36,* 503–12.

Paulson, M. J., and Wood, K. R. (1966). Perceptions of the emotional correlate of dysmenorrhea. *American Journal of Obstetrics and Gynecology, 95,* 991–96.

Perlmutter, J. F. (1978). A gynecological approach to menopause. In M. T. Notman and C. C. Nadelson (Eds.), *Sexual and Reproductive Aspects of Women's Health Care.* New York: Plenum.

Peskin, H. (1968). The duration of normal menses as a psychosomatic phenomenon. *Psychosomatic Medicine, 30,* 378–89.

Peyser, M. R., Ayalon, D., Harell, A., Toaff, R., and Cordova, T. (1973). Stress induced delay of ovulation. *Obstetrics and Gynecology, 42,* 667–71.

Phillips, N., and Duffy, T. (1973). One-hour glucose tolerance in relation to the use of contraceptive drugs. *American Journal of Obstetrics and Gynecology, 116,* 91–100.

Pierson, W. R., and Lockhart, A. (1963). Effect of menstruation on simple reaction and movement time. *British Medical Journal,* March, 796–97.

Plunkett, E. R., Moon, Y. S., Zamecnik, J., and Armstrong, D. T. (1975). Preliminary evidence of a role for prostaglandin F in human follicular function. *American Journal of Obstetrics and Gynecology, 123,* 391–95.

Pogmore, J. R., and Filshie, G. M. (1980). Flurbiprofen in the management of dysmenorrhoea. *British Journal of Obstetrics and Gynecology, 87,* 326–29.

Poliak, A., Smith, J. J., Friedlander, D., and Romney, S. L. (1971). Estrogen synthesis in castrated women: The action of human chorionic gonadotropin and corticotropin. *American Journal of Obstetrics and Gynecology, 110,* 376–79.

Polit, D. F., and LaRocco, S. A. (1980). Social and psychological correlates of menopausal symptoms. *Psychosomatic Medicine, 42,* 335–45.

Poller, L., Thomson, J. M., and Coope, J. (1980). A double-blind cross-over study of piperazine oestrone sulphate and placebo with coagulation studies. *British Journal of Obstetrics and Gynecology, 87,* 718–25.

Pontiroli, A. E., Baio, G., Stella, L., Crscenti, A., and Girardi, A. M. (1982). Effects of naloxone on prolactin, luteinizing hormone, and cortisol responses to surgical stress in humans. *Journal of Clinical Endocrinology and Metabolism, 55,* 378–80.

Porter, D. G., and Behrman, H. R. (1971). Prostaglandin-induced myometrial activity inhibited by progesterone. *Nature, 232,* 627–28.

Posner, J. (1979). It's all in your head: Feminist and medical models of menopause (strange bedfellows). *Sex Roles, 5,* 179–90.

Posner, N. A., Silverstone, F. A., and Tobin, E. H. (1975). Changes in carbohydrate tolerance during long-term oral contraception. *American Journal of Obstetrics and Gynecology, 123,* 119–27.

Preston, S. N. (1971). The oral contraceptive controversy. *American Journal of Obstetrics and Gynecology, 111,* 994–1007.

Price, J. M., Thornton, M. J., and Mueller, L. (1967). Tryptophan metabolism in women using steroid hormones for ovulation control. *American Journal of Clinical Nutrition, 20,* 452–56.

Pulkkinen, M. O. (1970). Regulation of uterine contractility. *Acta Obstetrica et Gynecologia Scandinavica, 49,* Supplement 1, 23–41.

Pulkkinen, M. O., Henzl, M. R., and Csapo, A. I. (1978). The effect of naproxen sodium on the prostaglandin concentrations of menstrual blood and uterine "jet-washings" in dysmenorrheic women. *Prostaglandins, 15,* 543–50.

Quigley, M. E., and Yen, S. S. C. (1980). The role of endogenous opiates on LH secretion during the menstrual cycle. *Journal of Clinical Endocrinology and Metabolism, 51,* 179–81.

Quillen, M. A., and Denney, D. R. (1982). Self-control of dysmenorrheic symptoms through pain management training. *Journal of Behavior Therapy and Experimental Psychiatry, 13,* 123–30.

Rader, M. D., Flickinger, G. L., de Villa, G. O., Mikuta, J. J., and Mikhail, G. (1973). Plasma estrogens in postmenopausal women. *American Journal of Obstetrics and Gynecology, 116,* 1069–73.

Rahe, R. H., Rubin, R. T., and Arthur, R. J. (1974). The three investigators study: Serum uric acid, cholesterol, and cortisol variability during stresses of everyday life. Psychosomatic Medicine, 36, 258–68.

Rakoff, A. E. (1975). Female climacteric: Premenopause, menopause, postmenopause. In J. J. Gold (Ed.), Gynecologic Endocrinology (2nd ed.). New York: Harper & Row.

Raz, S., Zeigler, M., and Adoni, A. (1971). Hormonal environment and uterine response to epinephrine. American Journal of Obstetrics and Gynecology, 111, 345–49.

Redmond, D. E., Murphy, D. L., Baulu, J., Ziegler, M. G., and Lake, C. R. (1975). Menstrual cycle and ovarian hormone effects on plasma and platelet monoamine oxidase (MAO) and plasma dopamine-beta-hydroxylase (DBH) activities in the rhesus monkey. Psychosomatic Medicine, 37, 417–28.

Rees, L. (1953). The premenstrual tension syndrome and its treatment. British Medical Journal, May, 1014–16.

Reeve, J., Tellex, M., Green, J. R., Hesp, R., Elsasser, U., Wootton, R., Hulme, P., Williams, D., Kanis, J. A., Russell, R. G. G., Mawer, E. B., and Meunier, P. J. (1982). Long-term treatment of osteoporosis with 24–25 dihydroxycholecalciferol. Acta Endocrinologica, 101, 636–40.

Reid, R. L., Hoff, J. D., and Yen, S. S. C. (1981). Effects of exogenous B-endorphin on pituitary hormone secretion and its disappearance rate in normal human subjects. Journal of Clinical Endocrinology and Metabolism, 52, 1179–84.

Reid, R. L., and Yen, S. S. C. (1981). Premenstrual syndrome. American Journal of Obstetrics and Gynecology, 139, 85–104.

—— (1983). The premenstrual syndrome. Clinical Obstetrics and Gynecology, 26, 710–18.

Resnik, R. (1981). The endocrine regulation of uterine blood flow in the nonpregnant uterus: A review. American Journal of Obstetrics and Gynecology, 140, 151–55.

Resnik, R., and Brink, F. W. (1980). Uterine vascular response to prostacyclin in nonpregnant sheep. American Journal of Obstetrics and Gynecology, 137, 267–69.

Resnik, R., Killam, A. P., Barton, M. D., Battaglia, F. C., Makowski, E. L., and Meschia, G. (1976). The effect of various vasoactive compounds upon the uterine vascular bed. *American Journal of Obstetrics and Gynecology, 125,* 201–6.

Reyes, F. I., Winter, J. S. D., and Faiman, C. (1977). Pituitary–ovarian relationships preceding the menopause. I. A cross-sectional study of serum follicle-stimulating hormone, luteinizing hormone, prolactin, estradiol, and progesterone levels. *American Journal of Obstetrics and Gynecology, 129,* 557–64.

Reynolds, S. R., Kaminester, S., Foster, F. L., and Schloss, S. (1941). Psychogenic and somatogenic factors in the flushes of the surgical menopause. *American Journal of Obstetrics and Gynecology, 41,* 1022–29.

Rigg, L. A., Milanes, B., Villaneuva, B., and Yen, S. S. C. (1977). Efficacy of intravaginal and intranasal administration of micronized estradiol-17B. *Journal of Clinical Endocrinology and Metabolism, 45,* 1261–64.

Riggs, B. L., Jowsey, J., Kelly, P. J., Hoffman, D. L., and Arnaud, C. D. (1976). Effects of oral therapy with calcium and vitamin D in primary osteoporosis. *Journal of Clinical Endocrinology and Metabolism, 42,* 1139–44.

Riggs, B. L., Ryan, R. J., Wahner, H. W., Jiang, K., and Mattox, V. R. (1973). Serum concentrations of estrogen, testosterone and gonadotropins in osteoporotic and nonosteoporotic postmenopausal women. *Journal of Clinical Endocrinology and Metabolism, 36,* 1097–99.

Robert, J. F., Quigley, M. E., and Yen, S. S. C. (1981). Endogenous opiates modulate pulsatile luteinizing hormone release in humans. *Journal of Clinical Endocrinology and Metabolism, 52,* 583–85.

Rodin, J. (1976). Menstruation, reattribution, and competence. *Journal of Personality and Social Psychology, 33,* 345–53.

Rogers, F. S. (1950). Emotional factors in gynecology. *American Journal of Obstetrics and Gynecology, 59,* 321–27.

Rogers, J. (1956). The menopause. *New England Journal of Medicine, 254,* 697–704.

Rogers, M. L., and Harding, S. S. (1981). Retrospective and daily menstrual distress measures in men and women using Moos' instruments (Forms A and T) and modified versions of Moos' instruments. In P. Komnenich, M. McSeeney, J. A. Noack, and N. Elder. (Eds.), *The Menstrual Cycle, Volume 2: Research & Implications for Women's Health.* New York: Springer Publishing.

Rolland, P. H., Martin, P. M., Rolland, A. M., Bourry, M., and Serment, H. (1979). Benign breast disease: Studies of prostaglandin E$_2$ steroids, and thermographic effects of inhibitors of prostaglandin biosynthesis. *Obstetrics and Gynecology, 54,* 715–18.

Rose, D. P. (1972). Aspects of tryptophan metabolism in health and disease: A review. *Journal of Clinical Pathology, 25,* 17–25.

Rose, D. P., and Adams, P. W. (1972). Oral contraceptives and tryptophan metabolism: Effects of oestrogen in low dose combined with a progestagen and a low-dose progestagen (megestrol acetate) given alone. *Journal of Clinical Pathology, 25,* 252–58.

Rose, D. P., Strong, R., Adams, P. W., and Harding, P. E. (1972). Experimental vitamin B$_6$ deficiency and the effect of oestrogen-containing oral contraceptives on tryptophan metabolism and vitamin B$_6$ requirements. *Clinical Science, 42,* 465–77.

Rosenblum, N. G., and Schlaff, S. (1976). Gonadotropin-releasing hormone radioimmunoassay and its measurement in normal human plasma, secondary amenorrhea, and postmenopausal syndrome. *American Journal of Obstetrics and Gynecology, 124,* 340–47.

Rosenwaks, Z., Jones, G. S., Henzl, M. R., Dubin, N. H., Ghodgaonkar, R. B., and Hoffman, S. (1981). Naproxen sodium, aspirin, and placebo in primary dysmenorrhea. *American Journal of Obstetrics and Gynecology, 140,* 592–98.

Rosenwaks, Z., Wentz, A. C., Jones, G. S., Urban, M. D., Lee, P. A., Migeon, C. J., Parmley, T. H., and Woodruff, J. D. (1979). Endometrial pathology and estrogens. *Obstetrics and Gynecology, 53,* 403–10.

Rosner, J. M., Nagle, C. A., de Laborde, M. P., Pedroza, E., Badano, A., Figueroa Casas, P. R., and Carril, M. (1976). Plasma levels of norepinephrine (NE) during the periovulatory period and after LH–RH stimulation in women. *American Journal of Obstetrics and Gynecology, 124,* 567–72.

Ross, R. K., Paganini-Hill, A., Gerkins, V. R., Mack, T. M., Pfeffer, R., Arthur, M., and Henderson, B. E. (1980). A case-control study of menopausal estrogen therapy and breast cancer. *Journal of the American Medical Association, 243,* 1635–39.

Rouse, P. (1978). Premenstrual tension: A study using the Moos Menstrual Questionnaire. *Journal of Psychosomatic Research, 22,* 215–22.

Roy, S. (1983). A double-blind comparison of a propionic acid derivative (ibuprofen) and a fenamate (mefenamic acid) in the treatment of dysmenorrhea. *Obstetrics and Gynecology, 61*, 628–32.

Ruble, D. N. (1977). Premenstrual symptoms: A reinterpretation. *Science, 197*, 291–92.

Ruble, D. N., and Brooks-Gunn, J. (1979). Menstrual symptoms: A social cognition analysis. *Journal of Behavioral Medicine, 2*, 171–94.

—— (1982). Expectations regarding menstrual symptoms: Effects on evaluation and behavior of women. In A. M. Voda, M. Dinnerstein, and S. R. O'Connell, *Changing Perspectives on Menopause*. Austin: University of Texas Press.

Sachar, E. J. (1980). Hormonal changes in stress and mentalillness. In D. T. Krieger and J. C. Hughes (Eds.), *Neuroendocrinology*. Sunderland, Mass.: Sinauer Associates, Inc.

Sakamoto, S., Satoh, K., and Kinoshita, K. (1976). Recent advances in prostaglandin research. In A. C. de Paz, V. A. Drill, M. Hayashi, W. Rodrigues, and A. V. Schally, *Recent Advances in Human Reproduction*. Amsterdam: Excerpta Medica.

Sanyal, M. K., Berger, M. J., Thompson, I. E., Taymor, M. L., and Horne, H. W. (1974). Development of graafian follicles in adult human ovary. I. Correlation of estrogen and progesterone concentration in antral fluid with growth of follicles. *Journal of Clinical Endocrinology and Metabolism, 38*, 828–35.

Sato, T., Jyujyo, T., Kawarai, Y., and Asai, T. (1975). Changes in LH-releasing hormone content of hypothalamus and electron microscopy of the anterior pituitary after prostaglandin E_2 injection in rats. *American Journal of Obstetrics and Gynecology, 122*, 637–41.

Sato, T., Taya, K., Jyujyo, T., Hirono, M., and Igarashi, M. (1974). The stimulatory effect of prostaglandins on luteinizing hormone release. *American Journal of Obstetrics and Gynecology, 118*, 875–76.

Schacter, S., and Singer, J. E. (1962). Cognitive, social, physiological determinants of motional state. *Psychological Review, 69*, 379–99.

Schally, A. V., Arimura, A., and Kastin, A. J. (1973). Hypothalamic regulatory hormones. *Science, 179*, 341–49.

Schilling, K. M. (1981). What is a real difference? Content or method in menstrual findings. In P. Komnenich, M. McSweeney, J. A. Noack, and

N. Elder (Eds.), The Menstrual Cycle, Volume 2: Research & Implications for Women's Health. New York: Springer Publishing.

Schinfeld, J. S., Tulchinsky, D., Schiff, I., and Fishman, J. (1980). Suppression of prolactin and gonadotropin secretion in post-menopausal women by 2-hydroxyestrone. Journal of Clinical Endocrinology and Metabolism, 50, 408–10.

Schmidt-Gollwitzer, M., Eiletz, J., Genz, T., and Pollow, K. (1979). Determination of estradiol, estrone, and progesterone in serum and myometrium: Correlation with the content of sex steroid receptors and 17B-hydroxy-steroid dyhydrogenase activity throughout the menstrual cycle. Journal of Clinical Endocrinology and Metabolism, 49, 370–76.

Schrotenboer, K., and Subark-Sharpe, G. J. (1981). Freedom from Menstrual Cramps. New York: Pocket Books.

Schuckit, M. A., Daly, V., Herrman, G., and Hineman, S. (1975). Premenstrual symptoms and depression in a university population. Diseases of the Nervous System, 36, 516–17.

Schwartz, A., Zor, U., Lindner, H. R., and Naor, S. (1974). Primary dysmenorrhea: Alleviation by an inhibitor of prostaglandin synthesis and action. Obstetrics and Gynecology, 44, 709–12.

Schwartz, U. D., and Abraham, G. E. (1975). Corticosterone and aldosterone levels during the menstrual cycle. Obstetrics and Gynecology, 45, 339–42.

Seligman, M. E. P. (1975). Helplessness. San Francisco: W. H. Freeman.

Selye, H. (1950). Stress: General-Adaptation Syndrome and the Disease of Adaptation. Montreal: ACTA, Inc.

Severne, L. (1982). Psychosocial aspects of the menopause. In A. M. Voda, M. Dinnerstein, and S. R. O'Connell, Changing Perspectives on Menopause. Austin: University of Texas Press.

Seyler, L. E., and Reichlin. S. (1973). Luteinizing hormone-releasing factor (LRF) in plasma of postmenopausal women. Journal of Clinical Endocrinology and Metabolism, 37, 197–203.

Sheldrake, P., and Cormack, M. (1976). Variations in menstrual cycle symptom reporting. Journal of Psychosomatic Research, 20, 169–77.

Sherman, L. M., West, J. H., and Korenman, S. G. (1976). The menopausal transition: Analysis of LH, FSH, estradiol, and progesterone concentrations during menstrual cycles of older women. *Journal of Clinical Endocrinology and Metabolism, 42,* 629–36.

Silbergeld, S., Brast, N., and Noble, E. P. (1971). The menstrual cycle: A double-blind study of symptoms, mood, and behavior, and biochemical variables using Enovid and placebo. *Psychosomatic Medicine, 33,* 411–28.

Simon, J. A., and di Zerega, G. S. (1982). Physiologic estradiol replacement following oophorectomy: Failure to maintain precastration gonadotropin levels. *Obstetrics and Gynecology, 59,* 511–13.

Singer, K., Cheng, R., and Schou, M. (1974). A controlled evaluation of lithium in the premenstrual tension syndrome. *Journal of Psychiatry, 124,* 50–51.

Singh, E. J., Baccarini, I. M., and Zuspan, F. P. (1975). Levels of prostaglandins F_{2a} and E_2 in human endometrium during the menstrual cycle. *American Journal of Obstetrics and Gynecology, 121,* 1003–6.

Skinner, S. L., Lumbers, E. R., and Symonds, E. M. (1969). Alteration by oral contraceptives of normal menstrual changes in plasma renin activity, concentration and substrate. *Clinical Science, 36,* 67–76.

Slade, P., and Jenner, F. A. (1980). Performance tests in different phases of the menstrual cycle. *Journal of Psychosomatic Research, 24,* 5–8.

Smith, D. C., Prentice, R., Thompson, D. J., and Herrmann, W. L. (1975). Association of exogenous estrogen and endometrial carcinoma. *New England Journal of Medicine, 293,* 1164–67.

Smith, K. D., Rodriques-Rigdu, L. J., and Steinberger, E. (1981). Introductions and counterintroductions for therapy with estrogen, progesterone and oral contraceptives. In P. Komnenich, M. McSweeney, J. A. Noack, and N. Elder (Eds.), *The Menstrual Cycle, Volume 2: Research & Implications for Women's Health.* New York: Springer Publishing.

Smith, R. P., and Powell, J. R. (1982). Intrauterine pressure changes during dysmenorrhea therapy. *American Journal of Obstetrics and Gynecology, 143,* 286–89.

Smith, R. W., and Rizek, J. (1966). Epidemiologic studies of osteoporosis in women of Puerto Rico and Southeastern Michigan with special reference to age, race, national origin, and to other related or associated findings. *Clinical Orthopaedics, 45,* 31–48.

Smith, S. L. (1975). Mood and the menstrual cycle. In *Topics in Psychoen-docrinology*. New York: Grune & Stratton.

Smith, S. L., and Sauder, C. (1969). Food cravings, depression, and pre-menstrual problems. *Psychosomatic Medicine, 31,* 281–87.

Somerville, B. W. (1971). Daily variation in plasma levels of progesterone and estradiol throughout the menstrual cycle. *American Journal of Obstetrics and Gynecology, 111,* 419–26.

___ (1975). Estrogen-withdrawal migraine. *Neurology,* 239–44.

Sommer, B. (1972). Menstrual cycle changes and intellectual performance. *Psychosomatic Medicine, 34,* 263–69.

___ (1973). The effect of menstruation on cognitive and perceptual-motor behavior: A review. *Psychosomatic Medicine, 35,* 515–34.

___ (1978). Stress and menstrual distress. *Journal of Human Stress, 4,* 5–10, 41–47.

___ (1984). PMS in the courts: Are all women on trial? *Psychology Today,* August, 36–38.

Sotrel, G., Helvacioglu, A., Dowers, S., Scommegna, A., and Auletta, F. J. (1981). Mechanism of luteolysis: Effect of estradiol and prostaglandin F_{2a} on corpus luteum luteinizing hormone/human chorionic gonado-tropin receptors and cyclic nucleotides in the rhesus monkey. *American Journal of Obstetrics and Gynecology, 139,* 134–40.

Southam, A. L., and Gonzaga, F. P. (1965). Systemic changes during the menstrual cycle. *American Journal of Obstetrics and Gynecology, 91,* 142–65.

Southgate, J., Grant, E. C. G., Pollard, W., Pryse-Davies, J., and Sandler, M. (1968). Cyclical variations in endometrial monoamine oxidase: Corre-lation of histochemical and quantitative biochemical assays. *Biochemical Pharmacology, 17,* 721–26.

Sowers, J. R., Raj, R. P., Hershman, J. M., Carlson, H. E., and McCallum, R. W. (1977). The effect of stressful diagnostic studies and surgery on anterior pituitary hormone release in man. *Acta Endocrinologica, 86,* 25–32.

Spellacy, W. N., Buhi, W. C., and Birk, S. A. (1975). Effects of norethin-drone on carbohydrate and lipid metabolism. *Obstetrics and Gynecology, 46,* 560–63.

Spellacy, W. N., Buhi, W. C., Birk, S. A., and Van Arnan, J. B. (1982). Carbohydrate metabolism studies in women using Brevicon, a low-estrogen type of oral contraceptive, for one year. *American Journal of Obstetrics and Gynecology, 142*, 105–8.

Spellacy, W. N., Newton, R. E., Buhi, W. C., and Birk, S. A. (1973). Carbohydrate and lipid studies during six months' treatment with megestrol acetate. *American Journal of Obstetrics and Gynecology, 116*, 1074–78.

Speroff, L., and Ramwell, P. W. (1970). Prostaglandins in reproductive physiology. *American Journal of Obstetrics and Gynecology, 107*, 1111–30.

Sporrong, B., Clase, L., Owman, Ch., and Sjoberg, N. O. (1977). Electron microscopy of adrenergic, cholinergic, and "p-type" nerves in the myometrium and a special kind of synaptic contacts with the "smooth" muscle cells. *American Journal of Obstetrics and Gynecology, 127*, 811–17.

Stangel, J. J., Innerfield, I., Reyniak, J. V., and Stone, M. L. (1977). The effect of conjugated estrogens on coagulability in menopausal women. *Obstetrics and Gynecology, 49*, 314–16.

Stavraky, K. M., Collins, J. A., Donner, A., and Wells, G. A. (1981). A comparison of estrogen use by women with endometrial cancer, gynecologic disorders, and other illnesses. *American Journal of Obstetrics and Gynecology, 141*, 547–55.

Steiner, J., Cassar, J., Mashiter, K., Dawes, I., Fraser, T. R., and Breckenridge, A. (1976). Effects of methyldopa on prolactin and growth hormone. *British Medical Journal, 1*, 1186–88.

Steptoe, A. (1980). Stress and medical disorders. In S. Rachman (Ed.), *Contributions to Medical Psychology*. New York: Pergamon.

Stromberg, P., Forsling, M. L., Akerlund, M. (1981). Effects of prostaglandin inhibition on vasopressin levels in women with primary dysmenorrhea. *Obstetrics and Gynecology, 58*, 206–8.

Studd, J. W. W., Chakravarti, S., and Oram, D. (1977). The climacteric. In R. B. Greenblatt and J. Studd (Eds.), *The Menopause: Clinics in Obstetrics and Gynecology*, Vol. 4. London: Saunders.

Studd, J. W. W., Dubiel, M., Kakkar, V. V., Thom, M., and White, P. J. (1978). The effect of hormone replacement therapy on glucose tolerance clotting factors, fibrinolysis and platelet behavior in postmenopausal women. In I. D. Cooke (Ed.), *The Role of Estrogen/Progesterone in the Management of the Menopause*. Baltimore, Md.: University Park Press.

Stumpf, P. G., Maruca, J., Santen, R. J., and Demers, L. M. (1982). Development of a vaginal ring for achieving physiological levels of 17B-estradiol in hypoestrogenic women. *Journal of Clinical Endocrinology and Metabolism, 54,* 208–10.

Sturdee, D. W., Wade-Evans, T., Paterson, M. E. L., Thom, M., and Studd, J. W. W. (1978). Relations between bleeding pattern, endometrial histology, and oestrogen treatment in menopausal women. *British Medical Journal, 1,* 1575–77.

Sturgis, S. H. (1970). Primary dysmenorrhea: Etiology and management. In S. A. Sturgis and M. L. Taymor (Eds.), *Progress in Gynecology,* Vol. V. New York: Grune and Stratton.

Sturgis, S. H., and Albright, F. (1940). The mechanism of estrin therapy in the relief of dysmenorrhea. *Endocrinology, 26,* 68–72.

Sullivan, S. F., and Marshall, J. M. (1970). Quantitative evaluation of effects of exogenous amines on contractility of human myometrium in vitro. *American Journal of Obstetrics and Gynecology, 107,* 139–49.

Sundsfjord, J. A., and Aakvaag, A. (1970). Plasma angiotensin II and aldosterone excretion during the menstrual cycle. *Acta Endocrinologia, 64,* 452–58.

Swandby, J. R. (1981). A longitudinal study of daily mood self-reports and their relationship to the menstrual cycle. In P. Komnenich, M. McSweeney, J. A. Noack, and N. Elder (Eds.), *The Menstrual Cycle, Volume 2: Research & Implications for Women's Health.* New York: Springer Publishing.

Sweat, M. L., and Bryson, M. J. (1970). Comparative metabolism of progesterone in proliferative human endometrium and myometrium. *American Journal of Obstetrics and Gynecology, 106,* 193–201.

Sweeney, D. R., and Maas, J. W. (1979). Stress and noradrenergic function in depression. In R. A. Depue, *The Psychology of the Depressive Disorders: Implications for the Effects of Stress.* New York: Academic Press.

Tapia, H. R., Johnson, C. E., and Strong, C. G. (1973). Effect of oral contraceptive therapy on the renin–angiotensin system in normotensive and hypertensive women. *Obstetrics and Gynecology, 41,* 643–49.

Tasto, D. L., and Chesney, M. A. (1974). Muscle relaxation treatment for primary dysmenorrhea. *Behavior Therapy, 5,* 668–72.

Tataryn, I. V., Lomax, P., Meldrum, D. R., Bajorek, J. G., Chesarek, W., and Judd, H. L. (1981). Objective techniques for the assessment of postmenopausal hot flashes. *Obstetrics and Gynecology, 57,* 340–44.

Tataryn, I. V., Meldrum, D. R., Lu, K. H., Frumar, A. M., and Judd, H. L. (1979). LH, FSH, and skin temperature during the menopausal hot flash. *Journal of Clinical Endocrinology and Metabolism, 49,* 152–54.

Taymor, M. L., and Thompson, I. E. (1975). Endocrinology of the menstrual cycle. In M. L. Taymor and T. H. Greed (Eds.), *Progress in Gynecology,* Vol. VI. New York: Grune and Stratton.

Teitelbaum, S. L., Rosenberg, E. M., Richardson, C. A., and Avioli, L. V. (1976). Histological studies of bone from normocalcemic postmenopausal osteoporotic patients with increased circulating parathyroid hormone. *Journal of Clinical Endocrinology and Metabolism, 42,* 537–43.

Telner, J. I., Merali, Z., and Singhal, R. L. (1982). Stress controllability and plasma prolactin levels in the rat. *Psychoneuroendocrinology, 7,* 36–44.

Thom, M., Chakravarti, S., Oram, D. H., and Studd, J. W. W. (1977). Effect of hormone replacement therapy on glucose tolerance in postmenopausal women. *British Journal of Obstetrics and Gynecology, 84,* 776–84.

Thom, M., Collins, W. P., and Studd, J. W. W. (1981). Hormonal profiles in postmenopausal women after therapy with subcutaneous implants. *British Journal of Obstetrics and Gynecology, 88,* 426–33.

Thorneycroft, I. H., Mishell, D. R., Stone, S. C., Kharma, K. M., and Nakamura, R. M. (1971). The relation of serum 17-hydroxyprogesterone and estradiol-17B levels during the human menstrual cycle. *American Journal of Obstetrics and Gynecology, 111,* 947–51.

Thorneycroft, I. H., Sribyatta, B., Tom, W. K., Nakamura, M., and Mishell, D. R. (1974). Measurement of serum LH, FSH, progesterone, 17-hydroxyprogesterone and estradiol-17B levels at 4-hour intervals during the periovulatory phase of the menstrual cycle. *Journal of Clinical Endocrinology and Metabolism, 39,* 754–58.

Tjellegen, L., Christiansen, C., Jummer, L., and Larsen, H. E. (1983). Unchanged biochemical indices of bone turnover despite fluctuations in

1,25-dihydroxyvitamin D during the menstrual cycle. *Acta Endocrinologica, 102,* 476–80.

Tolis, G., Dent, R., and Guyda, H. (1978). Opiates, prolactin and the dopamine receptor. *Journal of Clinical Endocrinology and Metabolism, 47,* 200–3.

Tonks, C. M., Rack, P. H., and Rose, M. J. (1968). Attempted suicide and the menstrual cycle. *Journal of Psychosomatic Research, 11,* 319–23.

Tsafriri, A., Lindner, H. R., Zor, U., and Lamprecht, S. A. (1972). Physiological role of prostaglandins in the induction of ovulation. *Prostaglandins, 2,* 1–9.

Tsai, C. C., and Yen, S. S. C. (1971). Acute effects of intravenous infusion of 17B-estradiol on gonadotropin release in pre- and post-menopausal women. *Journal of Clinical Endocrinology and Metabolism, 32,* 766–71.

Tsang, B. K., and Ooi, T. C. (1982). Prostaglandin secretion by human endometrium in vitro. *American Journal of Obstetrics and Gynecology, 142,* 626–33.

Tuch, R. H. (1975). The relationship between a mother's menstrual status and her response to illness in her child. *Psychosomatic Medicine, 37,* 388–94.

Tulandi, T., Lal, S., and Kinch, R. A. (1983). Effect of intravenous clonidine on menopausal flushing and luteinizing hormone secretion. *British Journal of Obstetrics and Gynecology, 90,* 854–57.

Tyson, J. E., and Friesen, H. G. (1973). Factors influencing the secretion of human prolactin and growth hormone in menstrual and gestational women. *American Journal of Obstetrics and Gynecology, 116,* 337–87.

Utian, W. H. (1972). The mental tonic effect of oestrogens administered to oophorectomized females. *South African Medical Journal, 46,* 1079–82.

Utian, W. H., Katz, M., Davey, D. A., and Carr, P. J. (1978). Effect of premenopausal castration and incremental dosages of conjugated equine estrogens on plasma follicle-stimulating hormone, luteinizing hormone, and estradiol. *American Journal of Obstetrics and Gynecology, 132,* 297–302.

Van Orden, D. E., Swanson, J. A., Clancey, C. J., and Farley, D. B. (1977). Plasma prostaglandins in the normal menstrual cycle. *Obstetrics and Gynecology, 50,* 639–43.

Vara, P. (1970). The climacterium from the gynaecologist's point of view. *Acta Obstetrica et Gynecologia Scandinavica, 49,* Supplement 1, 47–55.

Vermeulen, A. (1976). The hormonal activity of the postmenopausal ovary. *Journal of Clinical Endocrinology and Metabolism, 42,* 247–53.

Vijayakumar, R., and Walters, W. A. W. (1981). Myometrial prostaglandins during the human menstrual cycle. *American Journal of Obstetrics and Gynecology, 141,* 313–18.

Voda, A. (1980). Pattern of progesterone and aldosterone in ovulating women during the menstrual cycle. In A. J. Dan, E. A. Graham, and C. P. Beecher (Eds.), *The Menstrual Cycle, Volume 1: A Synthesis of Interdisciplinary Research.* New York: Springer Publishing.

___ (1981). Alterations of the menstrual cycle: Hormonal and mechanical. In P. Komnenich, M. McSweeney, J. A. Noack, and N. Elder (Eds.), *The Menstrual Cycle, Volume 2: Research and Implications for Women's Health.* New York: Springer Publishing.

___ (1982). Menopausal hot flash. In A. Voda, M. Dinnerstein, and S. R. O'Connell, *Changing Perspectives on Menopause.* Austin: University of Texas Press.

Vogel, N., Broverman, D. M., and Klaiber, E. L. (1971). EEG responses in regularly menstruating women and in amenorrheic women treated with ovarian hormones. *Science, 172,* 388–91.

von Kaulla, E., Droegemueller, W., and von Kaulla, K. N. (1975). Conjugated estrogens and hypercoagulability. *American Journal of Obstetrics and Gynecology, 122,* 688–92.

Walker, A. M., and Hershel, J. (1980). Declining rates of endometrial cancer. *Obstetrics and Gynecology, 56,* 733–36.

Walter, S., and Jensen, H. K. (1977). The effect of treatment with estradiol and estriol on fasting serum cholesterol and triglyceride levels in postmenopausal women. *British Journal of Obstetrics and Gynecology, 84,* 869–72.

Watkins, L. R., and Mayer, D. J. (1982). Organization of endogenous opiate and nonopiate pain control systems. *Science, 216,* 1185–92.

Webster, S. (1980). Problems for diagnosis of spasmodic and congestive dysmenorrhea. In A. J. Dan, E. A. Graham, and C. P. Beecher (Eds.), *The Menstrual Cycle, Volume 1: A Synthesis of Interdisciplinary Research.* New York: Springer Publishing.

Webster, S., Martin, H. J., Uchalik, D., and Gannon, L. (1979). The Menstrual Symptom Questionnaire and spasmodic/congestive dysmenorrhea: Measurement of an invalid construct. *Journal of Behavioral Medicine, 2,* 1–19.

Weideger, P. (1977). *Menstruation and Menopause.* New York: Knopf.

Weiner, B. (1974). *Achievement Motivation and Attribution Theory.* Morristown, N.J.: General Learning Press.

Weiner, J. S., and Elmadjian, F. (1962). Excretion of epinephrine and norepinephrine in premenstrual tension. *Federation Proceedings, 21,* 184.

Weiss, J. M., Glazer, H. I., Pohorecky, L. A., Bailey, W. H., and Schneider, L. H. (1979). Coping behavior and stress-induced behavioral depression: Studies of the role of brain catecholamines. In R. A. Depue (Ed.), *The Psychobiology of the Depressive Disorders: Implication for the Effects of Stress.* New York: Academic Press.

Wentz, A. C., Rocco, L., and Jones, G. S. (1975). Effect of PGF_{2a} in pseudopregnancy. *Obstetrics and Gynecology, 45,* 49–55.

Wetzel, R. D., McClure, J. N., and Reich, T. (1971). Premenstrual symptoms in self-referrals to a suicide prevention service. *British Journal of Psychiatry, 119,* 525–26.

Whitehead, M. I., McQueen, J., Minardi, J., and Campbell, S. (1978). Progestogen modification of estrogen-induced endometrial proliferation in climacteric women. In I. D. Cooke (Ed.), *The Role of Estrogen/ Progesterone in the Management of Menopause.* Baltimore, Md.: University Park Press.

Whitehead, R. E. (1934). Women pilots. *Journal of Aviation Medicine, 5,* 47–49. Cited in M. B. Parlee, The premenstrual syndrome. *Psychological Bulletin* (1973), *80,* 454–65.

Wickham, M. (1958). The effects of the menstrual cycle on test performance. *British Journal of Psychology, 49,* 34–41.

Wilcoxon, L. A., Schrader, S. L., Sherif, C. W. (1976). Daily self-report on activities, life events, moods, and somatic changes during the menstrual cycle. *Psychosomatic Medicine, 38,* 399–417.

Wilks, J. W., Wentz, A. C., and Jones, G. S. (1973). Prostaglandin F_{2a} concentrations in the blood of women during normal menstrual cycles and dysmenorrhea. *Journal of Clinical Endocrinology and Metabolism, 37,* 469–71.

Williams, A. R., Weiss, N. S., Ure, C. L., Ballard, J., Daling, J. R. (1982). Effect of weight, smoking, and estrogen use on the risk of hip and forearm fractures in postmenopausal women. *Obstetrics and Gynecology, 60,* 695–99.

Willman, E. A., Collins, W. P., and Clayton, S. G. (1976). Studies in the involvement of prostaglandins in uterine symptomatology and pathology. *British Journal of Obstetrics and Gynecology, 83,* 337–41.

Winston, F. (1969). Oral contraceptives and depression. *Lancet,* June, 1209.

Wong, W. H., Freedman, R. I., Levan, N. E., Hyman, C., and Quilligan, E. J. (1972). Changes in the capillary filtration coefficient of cutaneous vessels in women with premenstrual tension. *American Journal of Obstetrics and Gynecology, 114,* 950–53.

Wood, C., and Jakubowicz, D. (1980). The treatment of premenstrual symptoms with mefenamic acid. *British Journal of Obstetrics and Gynecology, 87,* 627–30.

Wood, K., and Coppen, A. (1978). The effect of estrogens on plasma tryptophan and adrenergic function in patients treated with lithium. In I. D. Cooke (Ed.), *The Role of Estrogen/Progesterone in the Management of the Menopause.* Baltimore, Md.: University Park Press.

Woods, N. F., Dery, G. K., and Most, A. (1982). Recollections of menarche, current menstrual attitudes and perimenstrual symptoms. *Psychosomatic Medicine, 44,* 285–93.

Woolf, P. D., Akowuah, E. S., Lee, L., Kelly, M., and Feibel, J. (1983). Evaluation of the dopamine response to stress in man. *Journal of Clinical Endocrinology and Metabolism, 56,* 246–50.

Woolf, V. (1929). *A Room of One's Own.* New York: Harcourt, Brace, and World.

World Health Organization: Task Force on Psychosocial Research in Family Planning (1981). A cross-cultural study of menstruation: Implications for contraceptive development. *Studies in Family Planning, 12,* 3–16.

Worley, R. J. (1981). Age, estrogen, and bone density. *Clinical Obstetrics and Gynecology, 24,* 203–18.

Wright, A. L. (1982). Variation in Navajo menopause: Toward an explanation. In A. M. Voda, M. Dinnerstein, and S. R. O'Connell (Eds.), *Changing Perspectives in Menopause.* Austin: University of Texas.

Wuttke, W., Arnold, P., Becker, D., Creutzfeldt, O., Langenstein, S., and Tirsch, W. (1975). Circulating hormones, EEG, and performance in psychological tests of women with and without oral contraceptives. Psychoneuroendocrinology, 1, 141–51.

Yen, S. S. C. (1980). Neuroendocrine regulation of the menstrual cycle. In D. T. Krieger and J. C. Hughes (Eds.), Neuroendocrinology. Sunderland, Mass.: Sinauer.

Yen, S. S. C., Martin, P. L., Burnier, A. M., Czekala, N. M., Greaney, M. O., and Callantine, R. (1975). Circulating estradiol, estrone, and gonadotropin levels following the administration of orally active 17B-estradiol in postmenopausal women. Journal of Clinical Endocrinology and Metabolism, 40, 518–21.

Ylikorkala, O., and Dawood, M. Y. (1978). New concepts in dysmenorrhea. American Journal of Obstetrics and Gynecology, 130, 833–47.

Ylikorkala, O., Puolakka, J., Kauppila, A. (1979). Serum gonadotrophins, prolactin, and ovarian steroids in primary dysmenorrhoea. British Journal of Obstetrics and Gynecology, 86, 648–53.

Ylostalo, P., Kauppila, A., Puolakka, J., Ronnberg, L., and Janne, O. (1982). Bromocriptine and norethisterone in the treatment of premenstrual syndrome. Obstetrics and Gynecology, 59, 292–98.

Young, M. M., and Nordin, B. E. C. (1967). Effects of natural and artificial menopause on plasma and urinary calcium and phosphorus. Lancet, July, 118–20.

Youngs, D. D., and Reame, N. (1983). Psychosomatic aspects of menstrual dysfunction. Clinical Obstetrics and Gynecology, 26, 777–84.

Zacur, H. A., Tyson, J. E., Ziegler, M. G., and Lake, C. R. (1978). Plasma dopamine-B-hydroxylase activity and norepinephrine levels during the human menstrual cycle. American Journal of Obstetrics and Gynecology, 130, 148–51.

Ziel, H. K., and Finkle, W. D. (1975). Increased risk of endometrial carcinoma among users of conjugated estrogens. New England Journal of Medicine, 293, 1167–70.

_____ (1976). Association of estrone with the development of endometrial carcinoma. American Journal of Obstetrics and Gynecology, 124, 735–40.

Zimmerman, E., and Parlee, M. B. (1973). Behavioral changes associated with the menstrual cycle. *Journal of Applied Social Psychology, 3*, 335–44.

Zuspan, F. P., and Zuspan, K. J. (1973). Ovulatory plasma amine (epinephrine and norepinephrine) surge in the woman. *American Journal of Obstetrics and Gynecology, 117*, 654–60.

INDEX

Name Index

Subject Index

About the Author

Linda Gannon is an Associate Professor of Psychology and the Director of Women's Studies at Southern Illinois University– Carbondale. She attended the University of Wisconsin–Madison where she received her doctorate in clinical psychology and psychophysiology in 1975. Dr. Gannon has published research articles in the areas of behavioral medicine and psychology of women and is co-editor, with Stephen Haynes, of *Psychosomatic Disorders: A Psychophysiological Approach to Etiology and Treatment*, published in 1981.